TYPE 2 DIABETES COOKBOOOK FOR BEGINNERS

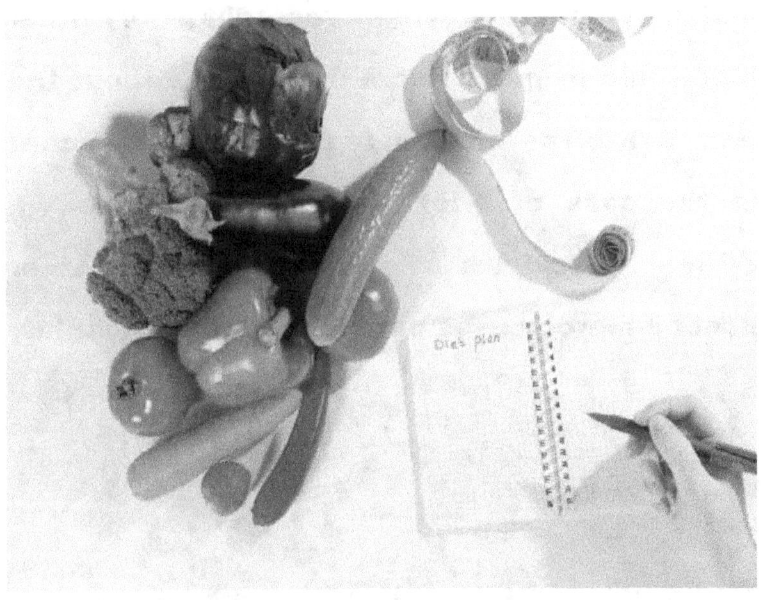

Simple, Tasty, and Healthy Low-Carb Recipes to Control Blood Sugar and Enhance Health

Rebecca T. Cook

Copyright © Rebecca T. Cook 2023

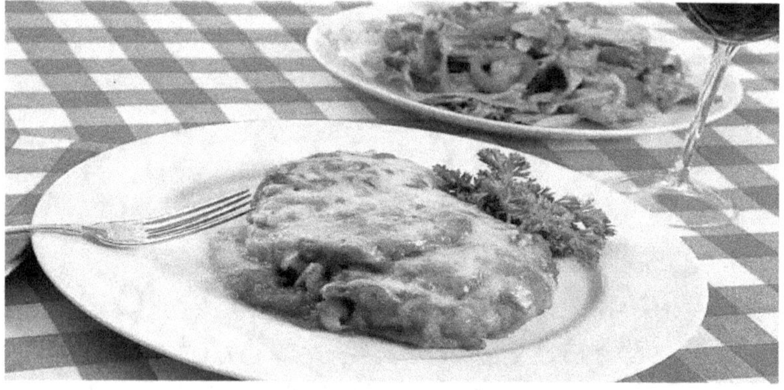

TABLE OF CONTENTS

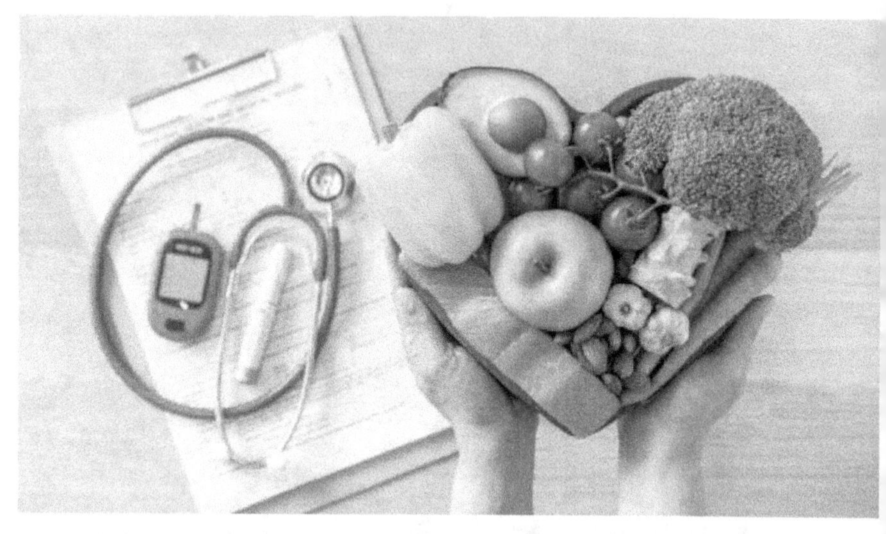

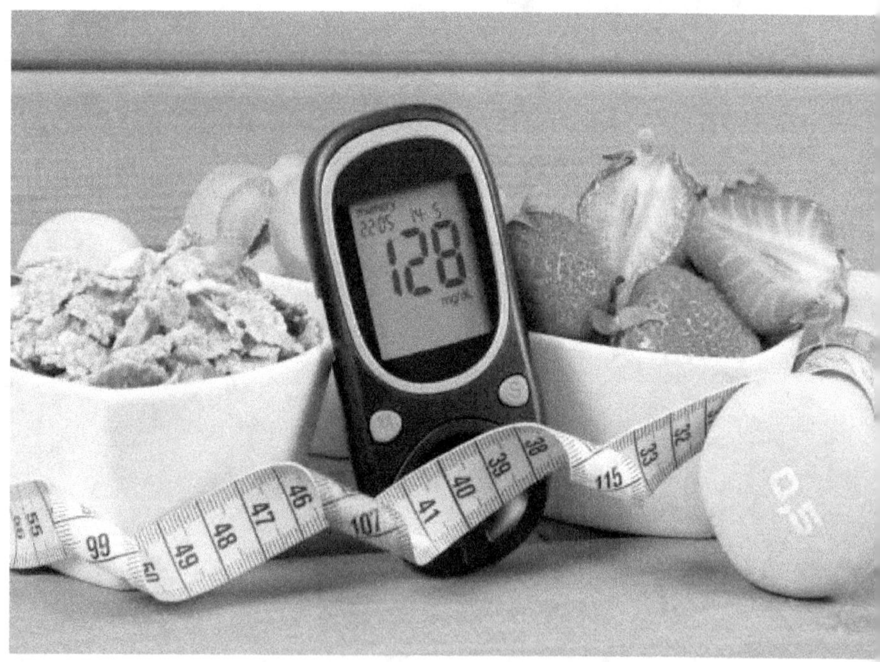

Introduction

Overview of Type 2 Diabetes

What then is Type 2 Diabetes?

Chronic type 2 diabetes affects how your body uses glucose, or sugar, which is an essential source of energy for your cells. Type 2 diabetes happens when the body develops resistant to insulin or when the pancreas is unable to create enough insulin to maintain normal glucose levels, in contrast to Type 1 diabetes, which is caused by the body's inability to make insulin. Elevated blood sugar levels result from this, and these can eventually lead to major health issues.

The   Effect   on   Well-being

Managing elevated blood sugar levels is not the only issue that comes with having Type 2 diabetes. It's a disorder that may have an impact on all facets of your life, emotionally and physically. Diabetes is a journey that frequently combines optimism, frustration, and dread. Fear stemming from uncertainty, possible problems, and a sense of powerlessness over one's health. annoyance at the ongoing observation, dietary limitations, and way of life adjustments. Nevertheless, despite these obstacles, there is hope: the prospect of a healthy future achieved by sensible management and lifestyle changes.

The consequences of uncontrolled Type 2 diabetes on long-term health are significant. Numerous issues, such as the following, can result from high blood sugar:

Cardiovascular disease: Elevated blood pressure, heart attack, and stroke risk.

Nerve Damage (Neuropathy): Usually affecting the extremities, this condition causes pain, tingling, and loss of feeling.

Nephropathy, or kidney damage; may lead to renal failure or the requirement for dialysis.

Retinopathy, or eye damage; increases the chance of blindness and other visual issues.

Foot Damage: Severe infections and even amputation can result from impaired blood flow and nerve damage.

Skin Conditions: Increased vulnerability to skin diseases and infections.

Type 2 diabetes can have negative effects on your mental and emotional health in addition to physical health. Stress, anxiety, and despair might result from the ongoing attention needed to treat the disease. Although it's a daily struggle, one that can be won with the correct information and resources.

Diet is Crucial for Managing Type 2 Diabetes

A key component of controlling Type 2 diabetes is diet. Your blood sugar levels might rise out of control or remain under control depending on what you consume. Adopting a nutritious, balanced diet is about empowerment as much as it is about limitation. It's about choosing foods that support your body, control your blood sugar, and improve your general health.

Whole meals such as fruits, vegetables, lean meats, and whole grains give vital elements that support stable blood sugar levels. Slow-digesting meals with a low glycemic index can help avoid blood sugar rises. While healthy fats can enhance insulin sensitivity, foods high in fiber can assist control the absorption of glucose.

Dietary management of Type 2 diabetes entails more than just cutting off sugar. It all comes down to knowing how various meals impact your body and making decisions that will help you reach your health objectives. It's about discovering happiness in new tastes and recipes that uplift your   spirits   within.

This cookbook is going to be your travel buddy. It is intended to present you with scrumptious, diabetes-friendly recipes that will empower you to take charge of your health in addition to tasting fantastic. Each dish is thoughtfully created with the specific dietary requirements of people with Type 2 diabetes in mind. Allow this book to serve as your road map to a more contented, joyful, and healthy existence.

Never forget that you are not traveling alone. You have the ability to improve your health with each and every meal. Accept the opportunities, enjoy the tastes, and manage your diabetes with optimism and confidence.

Nutritional Guidelines for Managing Type 2 Diabetes

To effectively manage Type 2 diabetes, you need to adopt a holistic approach to your health, where every food matters, rather than just taking your prescription and monitoring your blood sugar levels. The foods you select to feed your body may be a very useful ally on your path to better health. Here are some important dietary recommendations to help you walk this journey with hope and confidence.

Accept Low-Glycemic Meals

Think of the steady rise and fall of your blood sugar levels like the tides in a peaceful ocean. Foods low in glucose assist to stabilize these waves, avoiding the spikes and crashes that might make you feel ill. Because these foods digest slowly, energy is released gradually. Consider them your reliable pals who are there for you no matter what.

Whole Grains: Opt for whole grains rather than their refined equivalents, such as brown rice, quinoa, and whole wheat. Because of their high fiber content, they aid in blood sugar stabilization.

veggies: Include non-starchy veggies such as bell peppers, broccoli, cauliflower, and leafy greens on your plate. They are rich in vital nutrients and low in calories. *Legumes:* Rich in fiber and protein, beans, lentils, and chickpeas keep you full and content without raising blood sugar levels.

The Emotional Connection

Every meal is a chance to take care of and appreciate oneself. It involves adopting a lifestyle that promotes your happiness and health rather than merely avoiding particular meals. Imagine yourself in a healthy, energetic state, free from the difficulties that come with uncontrolled diabetes. Every decision you make moves you closer to that better future.

This cookbook serves as a travel companion in addition to being a compilation of recipes. You'll discover new methods to feed your body and spirit with each page, all while preparing delectable, diabetes-friendly meals. One mouthful at a time, we can together traverse the route to improved health.

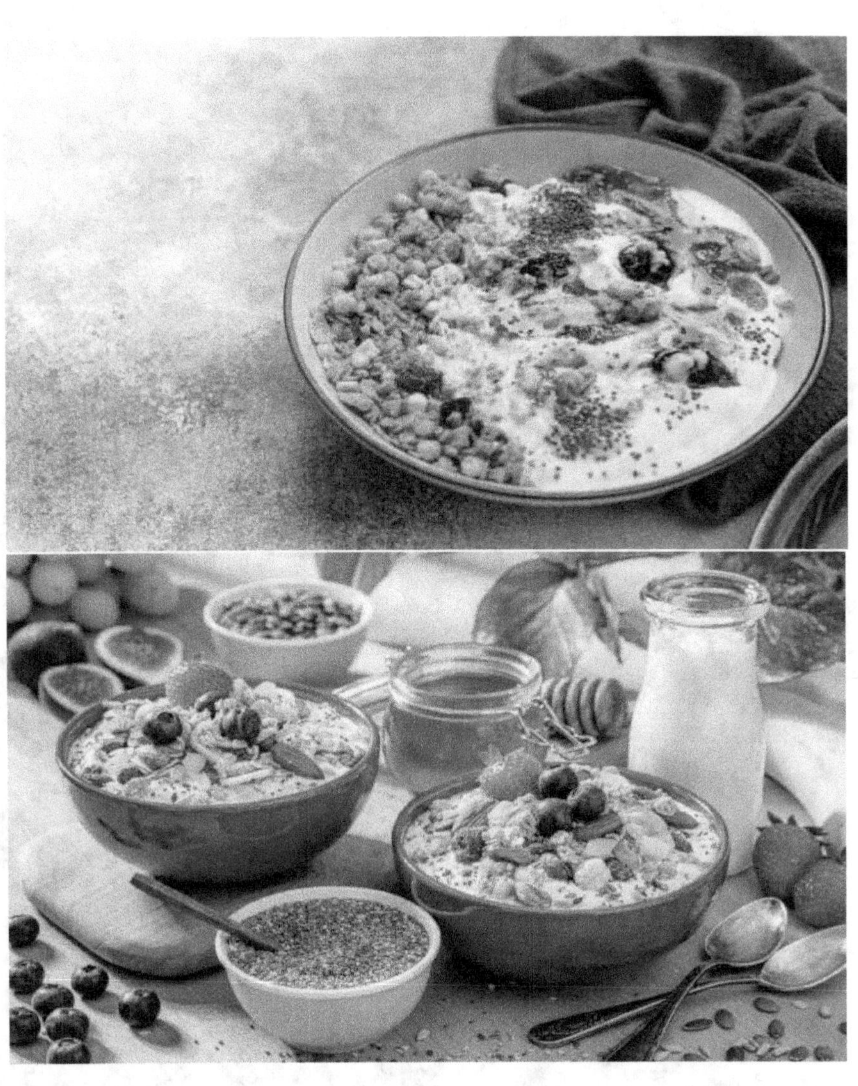

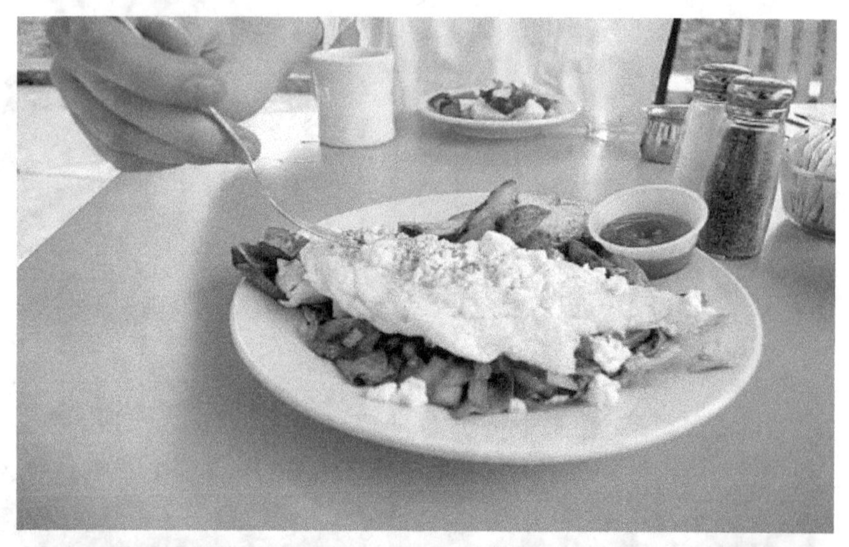

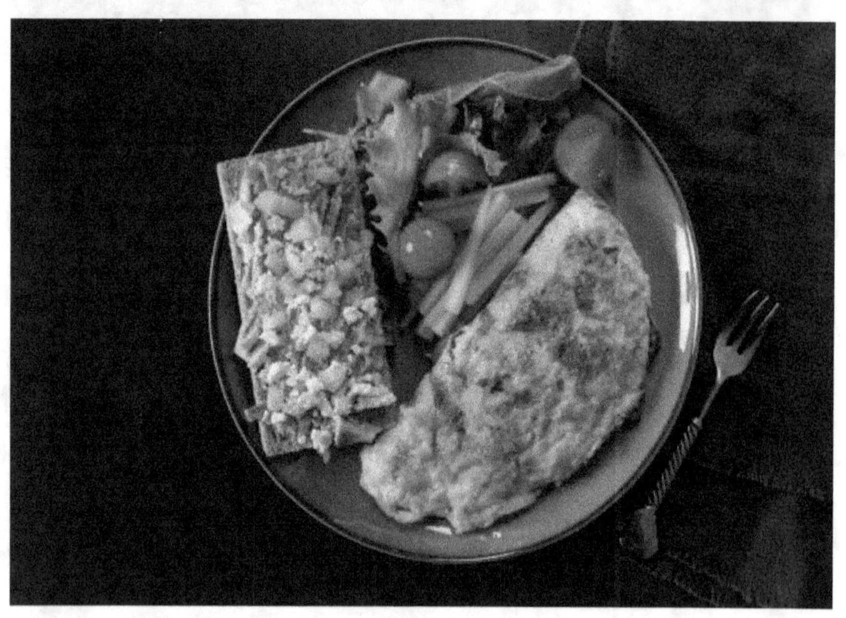

Chapter 1: Breakfast Recipes

1.Greek Yogurt with Chia Seeds and Berries

Ingredients:

- 1 cup Greek yogurt (plain, unsweetened)
- 1 tbsp chia seeds
- 1/2 cup mixed berries (blueberries, raspberries, strawberries)
- 1 tsp honey (optional)

Instructions:

- Combine chia seeds and Greek yogurt in a dish.
- Add a mixture of berries on top.
- If preferred, drizzle with honey.

Nutritional Values (per serving):

- Calories: 180
- Protein: 15g

- Carbs: 15g
- Fat: 6g
- Fiber: 6g

Health Benefits:

- Rich in protein to prolong feelings of fullness.
- Chia seeds include omega-3 fatty acids and fiber.
- Minimal in carbs and sugar.

2. Avocado and Egg Breakfast Bowl

Ingredients:

- 1 ripe avocado
- 2 eggs
- 1 tbsp olive oil
- Salt and pepper to taste
- 1/4 cup diced tomatoes
- 1 tbsp chopped cilantro

Instructions:

1. In a pan over medium heat, warm the olive oil.
2. Crack the eggs into the skillet and heat until they are cooked through.
3. Chop the avocado and transfer it to a bowl.
4. Add chopped cilantro, diced tomatoes, and fried eggs on top.
5. Add pepper and salt for seasoning.

Nutritional Values (per serving):

- Calories: 320
- Protein: 14g
- Carbs: 12g
- Fat: 28g
- Fiber: 10g

Health Benefits:

- Rich in protein and good fats.

- Avocado has important vitamins and fiber.

• Minimal in carbs, promoting steady blood sugar levels

3. Spinach and Feta Omelets

Ingredients:

- 3 large eggs
- 1/2 cup chopped fresh spinach
- 1/4 cup crumbled feta cheese
- 1 tbsp olive oil
- Salt and pepper to taste

Instructions:

1. Beat the eggs in a bowl and add pepper and salt to taste.
2. In a nonstick pan, warm the olive oil over medium heat.
3. Cook the spinach until it wilts.
4. Add the beaten eggs to the pan and heat them until they start to set.
5. Top the eggs with feta cheese.

Nutritional Values (per serving):

- Calories: 250
- Protein: 18g
- Carbs: 3g
- Fat: 19g
- Fiber: 1g

Health Benefits:

- Rich in good fats and protein.
- Vitamins, fiber, and iron are all found in spinach.
- Minimal in carbohydrates, ideal for controlling blood sugar.

4. Cottage Cheese with Nuts and Seeds

Ingredients:

- 1 cup cottage cheese (low-fat)
- 1 tbsp chopped almonds
- 1 tbsp sunflower seeds
- 1 tbsp pumpkin seeds

- 1/4 cup sliced strawberries

Instructions:

1. Put the cottage cheese, almonds, pumpkin seeds, and sunflower seeds in a dish.
2. Add sliced strawberries on top.

Nutritional Values (per serving):

- Calories: 220
- Protein: 20g
- Carbs: 10g
- Fat: 12g
- Fiber: 3g

Health Benefits:

• Rich in protein and healthy fats.

• Nuts and seeds offer minerals and fiber.

• Low in carbs, which helps regulate blood sugar.

5. Smoked Salmon and Avocado Toast

Ingredients:

- 1 slice whole-grain bread
- 1/2 avocado, mashed
- 2 oz smoked salmon
- 1 tsp lemon juice
- Salt and pepper to taste
- 1 tsp capers (optional)

Instructions:

1. Lightly toast the whole-grain bread piece.
2. Top the bread with avocado mash.
3. Add some smoked salmon on top.
4. Add a lemon juice drizzle and season with salt and pepper.
5. If you'd like, add capers.

- Calories: 280
- Protein: 15g
- Carbs: 20g
- Fat: 18g
- Fiber: 8g

Health Benefits:

• Properly proportioned with fiber, healthy fats, and protein.

• Omega-3 fatty acids are present in smoked salmon.

• Low in carbs, which helps control blood sugar levels.

6. Egg and Cheese Breakfast Muffins

Ingredients:

- 6 large eggs
- 1/2 cup shredded cheddar cheese
- 1/4 cup chopped bell peppers
- 1/4 cup chopped spinach
- Salt and pepper to taste

- 1 tbsp olive oil

Instructions:

1. Preheat oven to 350°F (175°C).
2. Grease a muffin tin with olive oil.
3. In a bowl, beat the eggs and season with salt and pepper.
4. Mix in cheese, bell peppers, and spinach.
5. Pour the mixture into the muffin tin.
6. Bake for 20-25 minutes or until the eggs are set.

Nutritional Values (per serving, 1 muffin):

- Calories: 110
- Protein: 8g
- Carbs: 2g
- Fat: 8g
- Fiber: 1g

Health Benefits:

- High in protein to keep you satisfied.
- Includes vegetables for added nutrients.

- Low in carbs, ideal for blood sugar control.

7. Protein Pancakes

Ingredients:

- 1 scoop protein powder (unsweetened, vanilla flavor)
- 1/2 cup almond flour
- 1/2 tsp baking powder
- 1/2 cup unsweetened almond milk
- 2 large eggs
- 1 tsp vanilla extract
- 1 tbsp coconut oil

Instructions:

1. In a bowl, combine protein powder, almond flour, and baking powder.
2. In another bowl, whisk together almond milk, eggs, and vanilla extract.
3. Mix wet ingredients into dry ingredients until smooth.

4. Heat coconut oil in a non-stick pan over medium heat.

5. Pour batter into the pan to form pancakes.

6. Cook until bubbles form, then flip and cook until golden brown.

Nutritional Values (per serving, 2 pancakes):

- Calories: 240
- Protein: 20g
- Carbs: 8g
- Fat: 14g
- Fiber: 3g

Health Benefits:

- High in protein, supports muscle maintenance.
- Almond flour is low in carbs and high in healthy fats.
- Suitable for a low-carb diet to manage blood sugar levels.

8. Chia Seed Pudding

Ingredients:

- 1/4 cup chia seeds
- 1 cup unsweetened almond milk
- 1/2 tsp vanilla extract
- 1 tbsp cocoa powder (optional)
- 1 tsp stevia or other sugar substitute (optional)

Instructions:

1. In a bowl, mix chia seeds, almond milk, and vanilla extract.
2. Add cocoa powder and stevia if desired.
3. Stir well and refrigerate overnight.
4. Serve chilled.

Nutritional Values (per serving):

- Calories: 150
- Protein: 6g
- Carbs: 12g

- Fat: 8g
- Fiber: 10g

Health Benefits:

- High in fiber and omega-3 fatty acids.
- Low in carbs and sugar.
- Supports digestive health and stable blood sugar levels.

9. Turkey Sausage and Egg Scramble

Ingredients:

- 2 turkey sausages, sliced
- 3 large eggs
- 1/4 cup diced bell peppers
- 1/4 cup diced onions
- 1 tbsp olive oil
- Salt and pepper to taste

Instructions:

1. In a pan over medium heat, warm the olive oil.

2. Cook the turkey sausage slices until they are browned.

3. Cook the onions and bell peppers until they are tender.

4. Beat the eggs in a bowl and add pepper and salt to taste.

5. Add the eggs to the skillet and heat until they are well scrambled.

Nutritional Values (per serving):

- Calories: 300
- Protein: 25g
- Carbs: 5g
- Fat: 20g
- Fiber: 2g

Health Benefits:

- High in protein to support muscle health.
- Low in carbs, beneficial for blood sugar management.
- Includes vegetables for added vitamins and minerals.

10. Tofu Scramble

Ingredients:

- 1 block firm tofu, crumbled
- 1/4 cup diced bell peppers
- 1/4 cup diced onions
- 1/4 cup spinach
- 1 tbsp olive oil
- 1 tsp turmeric
- Salt and pepper to taste

Instructions:

1. Heat the olive oil in a pan over medium heat.
2. Simmer the onions and bell peppers until they are soft.
3. Simmer the turmeric and tofu crumbles for five to seven minutes.
4. Cook until the spinach starts to wilt.
5. Season with salt and pepper.

Nutritional Values (per serving):

- Calories: 200
- Protein: 18g
- Carbs: 6g
- Fat: 12g
- Fiber: 4g

Health Benefits:

• Rich in protein, ideal for maintaining muscular mass.

• Low in carbohydrates, helps regulate blood sugar.

• Packed with antioxidants and phytonutrients from turmeric and veggies.

11. Cottage Cheese and Veggie Stuffed Peppers

Ingredients:

- 2 bell peppers, halved and seeds removed

- 1 cup low-fat cottage cheese

- 1/4 cup diced tomatoes

- 1/4 cup chopped cucumbers

- 1 tbsp chopped fresh parsley

- Salt and pepper to taste

Instructions:

1. Set oven temperature to 190°C/375°F.

2. Combine cottage cheese, chopped cucumbers, tomatoes, and parsley in a dish.

3. Add pepper and salt for seasoning.

4. Stuff the cottage cheese mixture into the bell pepper halves.

5. Arrange on a baking tray and cook for fifteen to twenty minutes.

Nutritional Values (per serving, 2 stuffed pepper halves):

- Calories: 180

- Protein: 20g
- Carbs: 10g
- Fat: 6g
- Fiber: 3g

Health Benefits:

- Rich in calcium and protein.
- Low in carbs, which helps regulate blood sugar.
- Contains veggies to provide extra nutrients and vitamins.

12. Almond Flour Waffles

Ingredients:

- 1 cup almond flour
- 2 large eggs
- 1/4 cup unsweetened almond milk
- 1 tbsp coconut oil, melted
- 1 tsp baking powder
- 1 tsp vanilla extract
- 1/4 tsp salt

1. Warm up your waffle maker.
2. Combine baking powder, salt, and almond flour in a bowl.
3. Beat eggs, coconut oil, almond milk, and vanilla extract in a separate dish.
4. Blend the ingredients, wet and dry, until smooth.

5. Fill the waffle iron with batter, and cook it till golden brown.

Nutritional Values (per serving, 2 waffles):

- Calories: 260
- Protein: 12g
- Carbs: 6g
- Fat: 22g
- Fiber: 4g

Health Benefits:

- Rich in good fats and protein.
- Low in carbs, which helps regulate blood sugar.
- Nutrients and fiber are found in almond flour.

13. Coconut Flour Pancakes

Ingredients:

- 1/4 cup coconut flour
- 3 large eggs
- 1/4 cup unsweetened almond milk
- 1 tsp vanilla extract
- 1/2 tsp baking powder
- 1 tbsp coconut oil

Instructions:

1. Combine eggs, almond milk, and vanilla essence in a bowl.
2. Blend in the baking powder and coconut flour until smooth.
3. In a nonstick pan, warm the coconut oil over medium heat.
4. Transfer batter into pan to make little pancakes.

5. Cook for 5 minutes, then turn and continue cooking until golden brown.

Nutritional Values (per serving, 2 pancakes):

- Calories: 180
- Protein: 10g
- Carbs: 8g
- Fat: 14g
- Fiber: 5g

Health Benefits:

- Rich in fiber and beneficial fats.
- Low in carbohydrates, making it perfect for controlling blood sugar.
- Coconut flour adds minerals and fiber.

14. Greek Yogurt Parfait with Nuts

Ingredients:

- 1 cup Greek yogurt (plain, unsweetened)
- 1/4 cup chopped walnuts
- 1/4 cup sliced almonds
- 1/4 cup mixed berries (blueberries, raspberries, strawberries)
- 1 tsp honey (optional)

Instructions:

1. Arrange berries, almonds, and Greek yogurt in a glass or dish.
2. Continue layering until all the ingredients have been utilized.
3. If desired, drizzle with honey.

Nutritional Values (per serving):

- Calories: 300
- Protein: 20g

- Carbs: 20g
- Fat: 18g
- Fiber: 6g

Health Benefits:

- Rich in protein to maintain fullness.
- Nuts offer fiber and good fats.
- Berries provide vitamins and antioxidants.

15. Egg White and Veggie Breakfast Wrap

Ingredients:

- 4 egg whites
- 1 whole-grain tortilla
- 1/4 cup chopped bell peppers
- 1/4 cup chopped spinach
- 1/4 cup diced tomatoes
- 1 tbsp olive oil

- Salt and pepper to taste

Instructions:

1. In a pan over medium heat, warm the olive oil.
2. Cook the tomatoes, spinach, and bell peppers until they are tender.
3. Beat the egg whites in a bowl and add pepper and salt to taste.
4. Add the egg whites to the skillet and heat them through to the center.
5. Fill the tortilla with the cooked vegetables and egg whites, then wrap.

Nutritional Values (per serving):

- Calories: 250
- Protein: 20g
- Carbs: 25g
- Fat: 8g
- Fiber: 6g

Health Benefits:

- Minimal fat and high protein content.
- Adds veggies for extra nutritional value.
- Whole-grain tortillas include fiber, which aids in improved digestion.

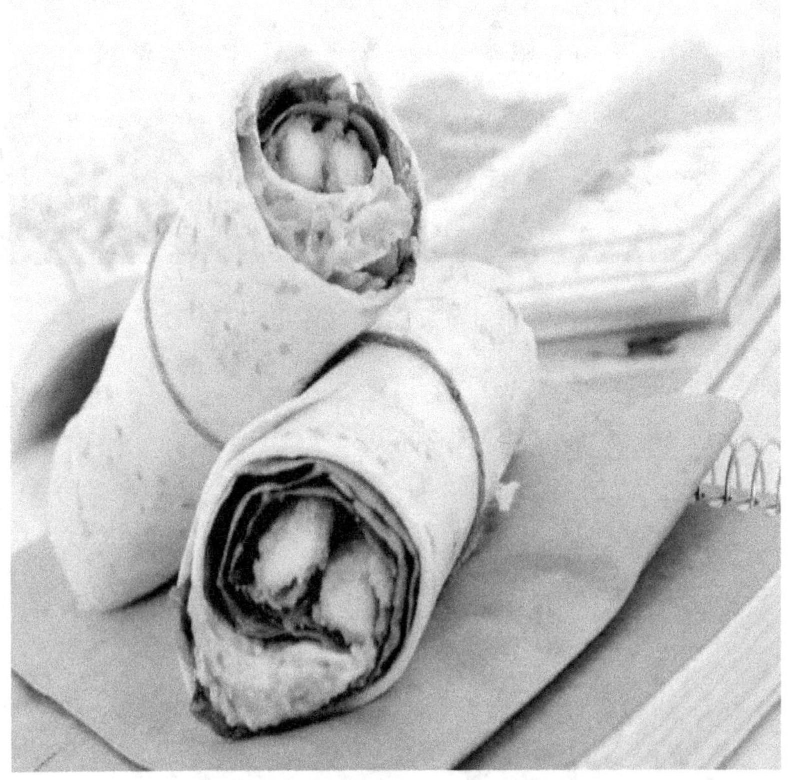

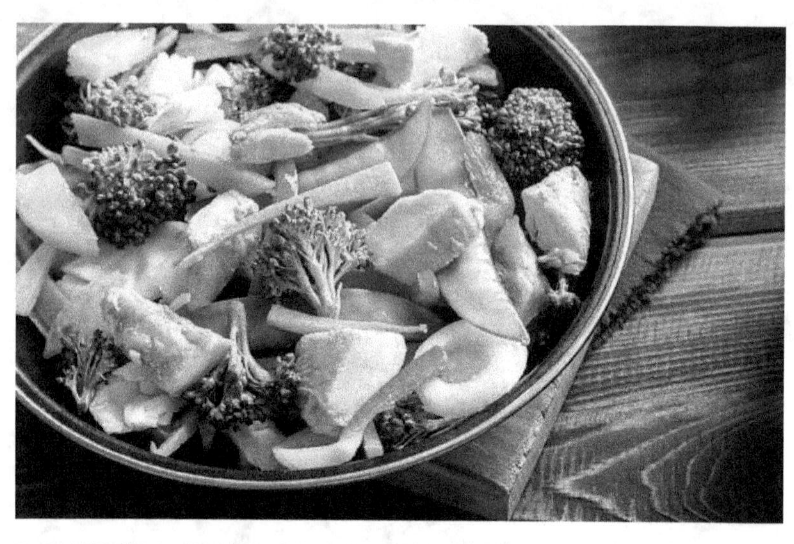

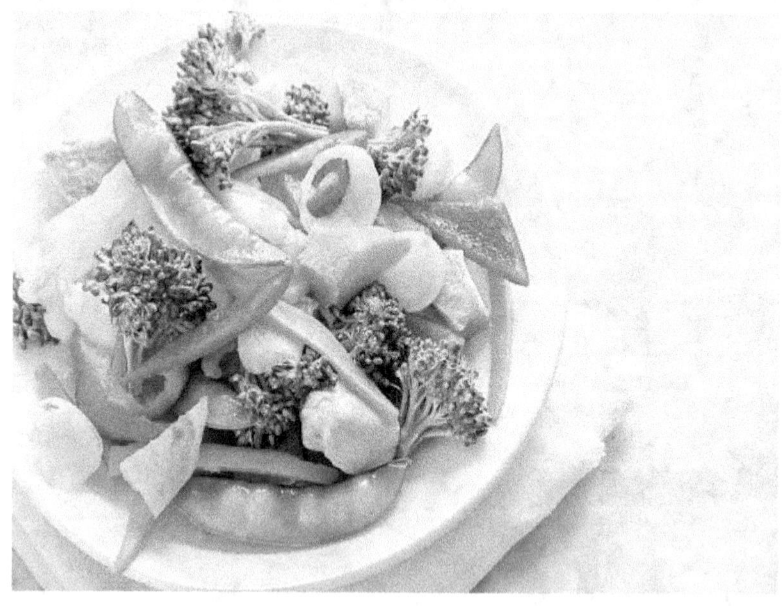

Chapter 2: Lunch Recipes

1. Grilled Chicken Salad

Ingredients:

- 1 grilled chicken breast, sliced
- 4 cups mixed greens
- 1/2 avocado, sliced
- 1/4 cup cherry tomatoes, halved
- 1/4 cup cucumber, sliced
- 2 tbsp olive oil
- 1 tbsp balsamic vinegar
- Salt and pepper to taste

Instructions:

1. Put the avocado, cherry tomatoes, cucumber, and mixed greens in a big bowl.
2. Arrange the cooked chicken slices on top.
3. Pour on some balsamic vinegar and olive oil.
4. Toss to mix after seasoning with salt and pepper.

Nutritional Values (per serving):

- Calories: 350
- Protein: 30g
- Carbs: 12g
- Fat: 22g
- Fiber: 8g

Health Benefits:

• Rich in good fats and protein.
• Low in carbohydrates, which helps with blood sugar control.
• Rich in antioxidants and vitamins from fresh veggies.

2. Tuna Salad Lettuce Wraps

Ingredients:

- 1 can tuna in water, drained
- 2 tbsp mayonnaise (preferably avocado or olive oil-based)
- 1 tbsp Dijon mustard
- 1/4 cup diced celery

- 1/4 cup diced red onion
- 4 large lettuce leaves
- Salt and pepper to taste

Instructions:

1. Combine tuna, red onion, celery, mayonnaise, and Dijon mustard in a bowl.
2. Use pepper and salt for seasoning.
3. Transfer the tuna salad to lettuce leaves, then wrap.

Nutritional Values (per serving, 2 wraps):

- Calories: 220
- Protein: 25g
- Carbs: 5g
- Fat: 12g
- Fiber: 2g

Health Benefits:

•Omega-3 fatty acids and protein content is high.
• Less carbohydrates, which is great for controlling blood

sugar.

• Water and fiber are found in lettuce.

3. Beef and Broccoli Stir-Fry

Ingredients:

- 1/2 lb lean beef, thinly sliced
- 2 cups broccoli florets
- 2 tbsp soy sauce (low-sodium)
- 1 tbsp olive oil
- 1 tsp minced garlic
- 1 tsp minced ginger
- 1/4 cup sliced green onions

Instructions:

1. In a large pan over medium-high heat, warm the olive oil.
2. Add the ginger and garlic, and cook until aromatic.
3. When the steak is cooked, add it.
4. Cook the broccoli until it is soft by adding it along with the soy sauce.
5. Add some green onions as a garnish and serve.

Nutritional Values (per serving):

- Calories: 300
- Protein: 30g
- Carbs: 10g
- Fat: 15g
- Fiber: 4g

Health Benefits:

• Rich in protein and low in carbohydrates.
• Contains cruciferous veggies, which are high in antioxidants and vitamins.
• Garlic and ginger contain anti-inflammatory qualities.

4. Turkey and Avocado Salad

Ingredients:

- 1 cup cooked turkey breast, shredded
- 1/2 avocado, diced
- 1/4 cup diced bell peppers
- 1/4 cup cherry tomatoes, halved

- 2 cups spinach leaves
- 2 tbsp olive oil
- 1 tbsp lemon juice
- Salt and pepper to taste

Instructions:

1. Combine turkey, avocado, cherry tomatoes, bell peppers, and spinach in a big bowl.
2. Add a lemon juice and olive oil drizzle.
3. Add salt and pepper to taste, then mix to blend.

Nutritional Values (per serving):

- Calories: 300
- Protein: 28g
- Carbs: 10g
- Fat: 18g
- Fiber: 6g

Health Benefits:

- Rich in good fats and protein.
- Minimal carbohydrates, which promote steady blood sugar

levels.

• Iron and important vitamins are found in spinach.

5. Salmon and Asparagus

Ingredients:

- 1 salmon fillet
- 1 bunch asparagus, trimmed
- 1 tbsp olive oil
- 1 tsp lemon zest
- 1 tsp garlic powder
- Salt and pepper to taste

Instructions:

1. Set oven temperature to 200°C/400°F.
2. Arrange the asparagus and fish on a baking sheet.
3. Add a drizzle of olive oil and season with salt, pepper, garlic powder, and lemon zest.
4. Bake for 15 to 20 minutes, or until the asparagus is soft and the salmon is cooked through.

- Calories: 350
- Protein: 30g
- Carbs: 10g
- Fat: 20g
- Fiber: 4g

Health Benefits:

- Rich in omega-3 fatty acids and protein.
- Low in carbohydrates, which helps regulate blood sugar.
- Asparagus has a lot of vitamins and fiber.

6. Chicken and Cauliflower Rice

Ingredients:

- 1 chicken breast, diced
- 2 cups cauliflower rice
- 1/2 cup diced bell peppers
- 1/4 cup diced onions
- 1 tbsp olive oil
- 1 tsp paprika

- 1 tsp garlic powder
- Salt and pepper to taste

Instructions:

1. In a pan over medium heat, warm the olive oil.
2. Cook the chicken until it becomes brown.
3. Cook the onions and bell peppers until they are tender.
4. Include the garlic powder, paprika, salt, pepper, and cauliflower rice.
5. Cook the cauliflower rice until it becomes soft.

Nutritional Values (per serving):

- Calories: 300
- Protein: 30g
- Carbs: 12g
- Fat: 16g
- Fiber: 6g

Health Benefits:

• Low in carbohydrates and high in protein.

• An option to grains that is low in carbs is cauliflower rice.

• Onions and bell peppers are good sources of vitamins and antioxidants.

7. Zucchini Noodles with Pesto and Shrimp

Ingredients:

- 2 cups zucchini noodles
- 1/2 lb shrimp, peeled and deveined
- 2 tbsp pesto sauce
- 1 tbsp olive oil
- 1 clove garlic, minced
- Salt and pepper to taste

Instructions:

1. In a pan over medium heat, warm the olive oil.

2. Cook the shrimp until they become pink by adding the garlic.

3. Add the zucchini noodles and simmer until soft, about 2 to 3 minutes.

4. Add the pesto sauce and season with pepper and salt.

Nutritional Values (per serving):

- Calories: 250
- Protein: 25g
- Carbs: 8g
- Fat: 14g
- Fiber: 4g

Health Benefits:

• Rich in good fats and protein.
• Minimal in carbohydrates, ideal for controlling blood sugar.
• Vitamins and fiber may be found in zucchini noodles.

8. Eggplant Lasagna

Ingredients:

- 1 large eggplant, sliced lengthwise
- 1 cup ricotta cheese
- 1 cup shredded mozzarella cheese
- 1/2 cup marinara sauce (no sugar added)
- 1/4 cup grated Parmesan cheese
- 1 egg
- 1 tsp Italian seasoning
- Salt and pepper to taste

Instructions:

1. Set oven temperature to 190°C/375°F.
2. Arrange the slices of eggplant and season with salt on a baking pan. After ten minutes of sitting, pat dry.
3. Combine the ricotta cheese, egg, salt, pepper, and Italian seasoning in a bowl.
4. Arrange the marinara sauce, mozzarella cheese, eggplant pieces, and ricotta mixture in a baking dish.
5. Continue layering and add Parmesan cheese on top.

6. Bake till bubbling and golden, about 30 to 35 minutes.

Nutritional Values (per serving):

- Calories: 320
- Protein: 22g
- Carbs: 15g
- Fat: 20g
- Fiber: 6g

Health Benefits:

- Rich in fiber and protein.
- Low in carbohydrates, which aids with blood sugar regulation.
- Vitamins and antioxidants may be found in eggplant.

9. Turkey Meatballs with Zoodles

Ingredients:

- 1 lb ground turkey
- 1/4 cup grated Parmesan cheese

- 1/4 cup almond flour

- 1 egg

- 2 cups zucchini noodles

- 1 cup marinara sauce (no sugar added)

- 1 tbsp olive oil

- 1 tsp Italian seasoning

- Salt and pepper to taste

Instructions:

1. Set oven temperature to 190°C/375°F.

2. Combine the ground turkey, egg, almond flour, Parmesan cheese, Italian seasoning, salt, and pepper in a basin.

3. Shape the mixture into meatballs and arrange them on a baking tray.

4. Bake for 20 to 25 minutes, or until well done.

5. Cook the zucchini noodles in hot olive oil in a pan until they are soft.

6. Place the meatballs and marinara sauce in the skillet and fully cook.

Nutritional Values (per serving):

- Calories: 350
- Protein: 30g
- Carbs: 12g
- Fat: 20g
- Fiber: 5g

Health Benefits:

• Rich in protein to promote the health of muscles.

• Low in carbs, which helps to regulate blood sugar.

• A fantastic low-carb substitute for pasta is zucchini noodles.

10. Spicy Chickpea and Avocado Salad

Ingredients:

- 1 can chickpeas, drained and rinsed
- 1 avocado, diced

- 1/4 cup diced red onion
- 1/4 cup chopped cilantro
- 1 jalapeño, seeded and diced
- 2 tbsp olive oil
- 1 tbsp lime juice
- 1 tsp cumin
- Salt and pepper to taste

Instructions:

1. Combine the avocado, red onion, cilantro, jalapeño, and chickpeas in a big bowl.
2. Combine the olive oil, lime juice, cumin, salt, and pepper in a small bowl.
3. Drizzle the salad with the dressing and mix thoroughly.

Nutritional Values (per serving):

- Calories: 350

- Protein: 12g
- Carbs: 30g
- Fat: 22g
- Fiber: 12g

Health Benefits:

- Rich in good fats and fiber.
- Moderate protein content for a full and substantial meal.
- Avocado offers vital nutrients and vitamins.

11. Stuffed Bell Peppers with Quinoa and Turkey

Ingredients:

- 4 large bell peppers, tops cut off and seeds removed
- 1 cup cooked quinoa
- 1/2 lb ground turkey
- 1/2 cup diced tomatoes
- 1/4 cup diced onions
- 1/4 cup shredded mozzarella cheese

- 1 tbsp olive oil
- 1 tsp Italian seasoning
- Salt and pepper to taste

Instructions:

1. Set oven temperature to 190°C/375°F.
2. Heat the olive oil in a pan and sauté the onions until they are transparent.
3. Add the turkey meat and heat it until it browns.
4. Add the diced tomatoes, cooked quinoa, salt, pepper, and Italian seasoning.
5. Stuff mixture into bell peppers and arrange in baking dish.
6. Add shredded mozzarella cheese on top.
7. Bake the peppers for 20 to 25 minutes, or until they are soft.

Nutritional Values (per serving, 1 stuffed pepper):

- Calories: 280
- Protein: 20g

- Carbs: 25g
- Fat: 12g
- Fiber: 6g

Health Benefits:

- Rich in fiber and protein.
- Quinoa offers all the necessary nutrients and complete protein.
- Low in carbohydrates, which helps regulate blood sugar.

12. Chicken and Avocado Lettuce Wraps

Ingredients:

- 1 chicken breast, cooked and shredded
- 1 avocado, diced
- 1/4 cup diced tomatoes
- 1/4 cup diced red onions
- 2 tbsp lime juice
- 1 tbsp chopped cilantro

- 4 large lettuce leaves
- Salt and pepper to taste

Instructions:

1. Combine the shredded chicken, avocado, lime juice, cilantro, tomatoes, and red onions in a bowl.
2. Add pepper and salt for seasoning.
3. Transfer the blend onto lettuce leaves and enclose.

Nutritional Values (per serving, 2 wraps):

- Calories: 250
- Protein: 20g
- Carbs: 8g
- Fat: 16g
- Fiber: 6g

Health Benefits:

- Rich in good fats and protein.
- Rich in fiber, perfect for controlling blood sugar levels.
- Lettuce offers hydration and fiber.

13. Beef and Avocado Salad

Ingredients:

- 1 cup cooked beef, sliced
- 1/2 avocado, sliced
- 4 cups mixed greens
- 1/4 cup cherry tomatoes, halved
- 1/4 cup cucumber, sliced
- 2 tbsp olive oil
- 1 tbsp balsamic vinegar
- Salt and pepper to taste

Instructions:

1. Put the cucumber, cherry tomatoes, avocado, and mixed greens in a big bowl.
2. Place sliced beef on top.
3. Drizzle with balsamic vinegar and olive oil.
4. Add salt and pepper, then toss to mix.

- Calories: 350
- Protein: 28g
- Carbs: 10g
- Fat: 22g
- Fiber: 8g

Health Benefits:

• Rich in good fats and protein.
• Minimal carbohydrates, which promote steady blood sugar levels.
• Rich in antioxidants and vitamins from fresh veggies.

14. Salmon and Avocado Bowl

Ingredients:

- 1 salmon fillet, cooked and flaked
- 1/2 avocado, sliced
- 1/4 cup shredded carrots
- 1/4 cup sliced cucumber

- 2 cups mixed greens
- 2 tbsp sesame seeds
- 1 tbsp olive oil
- 1 tbsp soy sauce (low-sodium)

Instructions:

1. Combine shredded carrots, sliced cucumber, and mixed greens in a big dish.
2. Place avocado slices and flaked salmon on top.
3. Add a dash of sesame seeds.
4. Add a soy sauce and olive oil drizzle.

Nutritional Values (per serving):

- Calories: 380
- Protein: 28g
- Carbs: 12g
- Fat: 26g
- Fiber: 8g

• Rich in omega-3 fatty acids and protein.

• Low in carbohydrates, which helps regulate blood sugar.

• Essential nutrients and fiber are found in fresh veggies.

15. Chicken and Broccoli Stir-Fry

Ingredients:

- 1 chicken breast, sliced
- 2 cups broccoli florets
- 1/4 cup diced onions
- 1 tbsp soy sauce (low-sodium)
- 1 tbsp olive oil
- 1 tsp garlic powder
- Salt and pepper to taste

Instructions:

1. In a pan over medium-high heat, warm the olive oil.
2. Cook the onions until they become tender.

3. Cook the chicken until it becomes brown.

4. Include the broccoli, salt, pepper, garlic powder, and soy sauce.

5. Sauté the broccoli until it's soft.

Nutritional Values (per serving):

- Calories: 300
- Protein: 28g
- Carbs: 10g
- Fat: 16g
- Fiber: 4g

Health Benefits:

- Low in carbohydrates and high in protein.
- Broccoli has antioxidants, vitamins, and fiber.
- Garlic powder enhances taste and may have health advantages.

16. Cabbage Roll-Ups with Ground Beef

Ingredients:

- 8 large cabbage leaves
- 1 lb ground beef
- 1/2 cup diced onions
- 1/2 cup diced tomatoes
- 1 tsp garlic powder
- 1 tsp paprika
- Salt and pepper to taste

Instructions:

1. Brown the ground beef and onions in a pan.
2. Add the diced tomatoes, paprika, garlic powder, salt, and pepper.
3. Blanch cabbage leaves for two minutes in boiling water, then remove.
4. Spoon each cabbage leaf with a heaping tablespoon of the meat mixture, then roll up.
5. You may serve right away or refrigerate for later.

Nutritional Values (per serving, 2 roll-ups):

- Calories: 250
- Protein: 20g
- Carbs: 10g
- Fat: 15g
- Fiber: 4g

Health Benefits:

- Low in carbohydrates and high in protein.
- Antioxidants and fiber are found in cabbage.
- An easy and wholesome dinner choice.

17. Shrimp and Avocado Salad

Ingredients:

- 1/2 lb cooked shrimp
- 1 avocado, diced
- 1/4 cup diced red bell pepper
- 1/4 cup diced cucumber

- 2 tbsp lime juice
- 1 tbsp olive oil
- Salt and pepper to taste

Instructions:

1. Combine the bell pepper, cucumber, avocado, and shrimp in a big bowl.
2. Add a drizzle of olive oil and lime juice.
3. Add salt and pepper to taste, then mix to blend.

Nutritional Values (per serving):

- Calories: 300
- Protein: 25g
- Carbs: 10g
- Fat: 18g
- Fiber: 6g

Health Benefits:

- Rich in good fats and protein.
- Minimal in carbohydrates, ideal for controlling blood

sugar.

• Avocado offers vital nutrients and vitamins.

18. Cauliflower Fried Rice with Chicken

Ingredients:

- 1 chicken breast, diced
- 2 cups cauliflower rice
- 1/2 cup diced carrots
- 1/2 cup peas
- 1/4 cup diced onions
- 2 eggs, beaten
- 2 tbsp soy sauce (low-sodium)
- 1 tbsp olive oil
- Salt and pepper to taste

Instructions:

1. In a pan over medium heat, warm the olive oil.

2. Cook the carrots and onions until they are tender.

3. Cook the chicken until it becomes brown.

4.   Transfer ingredients to one side while arranging the eggs on the other.

5. Combine all ingredients and stir in the peas, cauliflower rice, and soy sauce.

6. Cook the cauliflower rice until it becomes soft.

Nutritional Values (per serving):

- Calories: 350
- Protein: 28g
- Carbs: 15g
- Fat: 18g
- Fiber: 6g

Health Benefits:

• Rich in protein to maintain the health of muscles.

• Minimal carbohydrates, good for controlling blood sugar.

• A fantastic low-carb option to regular rice is cauliflower rice.

19. Greek Chicken Bowl

Ingredients:

- 1 chicken breast, grilled and sliced
- 1/2 cup cherry tomatoes, halved
- 1/2 cucumber, diced
- 1/4 cup red onion, thinly sliced
- 1/4 cup Kalamata olives, pitted and halved
- 2 cups mixed greens
- 2 tbsp crumbled feta cheese
- 2 tbsp olive oil
- 1 tbsp lemon juice
- 1 tsp dried oregano
- Salt and pepper to taste

Instructions:

1. Put mixed greens, cherry tomatoes, cucumber, red onion, and olives in a big bowl.
2. Add some crumbled feta cheese and cooked chicken on top.

3. Combine the olive oil, lemon juice, oregano, salt, and pepper in a small bowl.

4. Cover the salad with the dressing and toss to mix.

Nutritional Values (per serving):

- Calories: 350
- Protein: 28g
- Carbs: 12g
- Fat: 22g
- Fiber: 5g

Health Benefits:

- Rich in good fats and protein.
- Low in carbohydrates, which aids with blood sugar regulation.
- Antioxidants and vitamins are found in fresh veggies.

20. Baked Cod with Vegetables

Ingredients:

- 1 cod fillet
- 1/2 cup cherry tomatoes, halved
- 1/2 cup zucchini, sliced
- 1/2 cup yellow squash, sliced
- 2 tbsp olive oil
- 1 tbsp lemon juice
- 1 tsp dried thyme
- Salt and pepper to taste

Instructions:

1. Set oven temperature to 190°C/375°F.
2. Put the fillet of fish onto a baking sheet.
3. Arrange yellow squash, zucchini, and cherry tomatoes around the fish.
4. Drizzle with lemon juice and olive oil.
5. Add a dash of pepper, salt, and dry thyme.
6. Bake for 20 to 25 minutes, or until the veggies are soft and the fish is cooked through.

Nutritional Values (per serving):

- Calories: 250
- Protein: 25g
- Carbs: 10g
- Fat: 14g
- Fiber: 4g

Health Benefits:

• Rich in omega-3 fatty acids and protein.
• Minimal carbohydrates, which promote steady blood sugar levels.
• Fiber and important vitamins are found in vegetables.

21. Chicken and Spinach Stuffed Mushrooms

Ingredients:

- 4 large portobello mushrooms, stems removed

- 1 cup cooked chicken breast, shredded
- 1/2 cup cooked spinach, drained and chopped
- 1/4 cup ricotta cheese
- 1/4 cup shredded mozzarella cheese
- 1 clove garlic, minced
- Salt and pepper to taste

Instructions:

1. Set oven temperature to 190°C/375°F.
2. Combine the ricotta cheese, garlic, spinach, shredded chicken, salt, and pepper in a bowl.
3. Insert the mixture into the caps of the mushrooms.
4. Add shredded mozzarella cheese on top.
5. Bake for 20 to 25 minutes, or until the cheese has melted and the mushrooms are soft.

Nutritional Values (per serving, 2 stuffed mushrooms):

- Calories: 300
- Protein: 28g
- Carbs: 8g

- Fat: 18g
- Fiber: 4g

Health Benefits:

• Low in carbohydrates and high in protein.

• Iron, vitamins, and antioxidants are found in spinach.

• Mushrooms provide extra fiber and minerals.

22. Turkey and Cabbage Stir-Fry

Ingredients:

- 1/2 lb ground turkey
- 2 cups shredded cabbage
- 1/4 cup diced onions
- 1/4 cup diced bell peppers
- 1 tbsp soy sauce (low-sodium)
- 1 tbsp olive oil
- 1 tsp garlic powder
- Salt and pepper to taste

Instructions:

1. In a pan over medium heat, warm the olive oil.
2. Cook the bell peppers and onions until they are tender.
3. Add the turkey meat and heat it until it browns.
4. Include the soy sauce, salt, pepper, garlic powder, and chopped cabbage.
5. Cook the cabbage until it is soft.

Nutritional Values (per serving):

- Calories: 280
- Protein: 24g
- Carbs: 12g
- Fat: 14g
- Fiber: 5g

Health Benefits:

- Low in carbohydrates and high in protein.
- Vitamins and fiber are found in cabbage.
- One option for lean protein is ground turkey.

23. Pesto Chicken and Veggie Skewers

Ingredients:

- 1 chicken breast, cut into cubes
- 1/2 cup cherry tomatoes
- 1/2 zucchini, sliced
- 1/2 red bell pepper, cut into squares
- 1/4 cup pesto sauce
- 1 tbsp olive oil
- Salt and pepper to taste

Instructions:

1. Turn the heat up to medium-high on the grill or grill pan.
2. Thread bell pepper, zucchini, cherry tomatoes, and chicken onto skewers.

3. Use olive oil and pesto sauce to brush.

4. Add pepper and salt for seasoning.

5. Grill the skewers for ten to fifteen minutes, rotating them now and again, or until the chicken is well cooked and the veggies are soft.

Nutritional Values (per serving, 2 skewers):

- Calories: 320
- Protein: 28g
- Carbs: 8g
- Fat: 20g
- Fiber: 3g

Health Benefits:

- Rich in good fats and protein.
- Low in carbohydrates, which helps regulate blood sugar.
- Vitamins and antioxidants are found in vegetables.

24. Beef and Spinach Stuffed Peppers

Ingredients:

- 4 bell peppers, tops cut off and seeds removed
- 1/2 lb ground beef
- 1 cup cooked spinach, drained and chopped
- 1/2 cup diced tomatoes
- 1/4 cup shredded mozzarella cheese
- 1 tbsp olive oil
- 1 tsp Italian seasoning
- Salt and pepper to taste

Instructions:

1. Turn the oven on to 375°F, or 190°C.
2. Brown the ground beef in a pan with hot olive oil.
3. Add salt, pepper, Italian seasoning, cooked spinach, and diced tomatoes.
4. Place the bell peppers in a baking tray after stuffing them with the mixture.
5. Add mozzarella cheese shreds on top.

6. Bake for twenty to thirty minutes, or until peppers are soft.

Nutritional Values (per serving, 1 stuffed pepper):

- Calories: 280
- Protein: 22g
- Carbs: 15g
- Fat: 16g
- Fiber: 5g

Health Benefits:

- Low in carbohydrates and high in protein.
- Iron and other necessary nutrients are found in spinach.
- Antioxidants and vitamins abound in bell peppers.

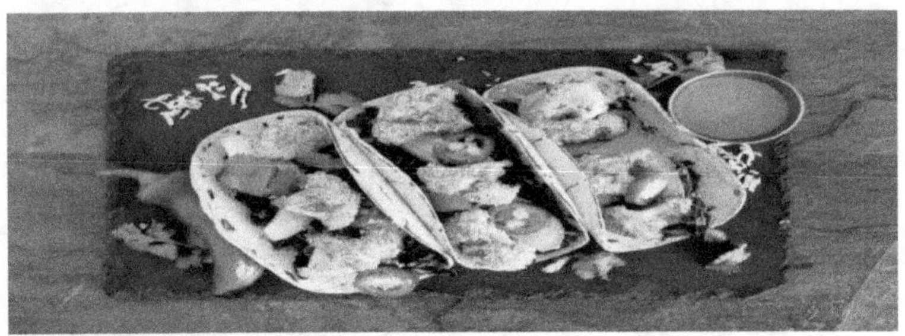

25. Grilled Steak Salad

Ingredients:

- 1 steak (about 6 oz), grilled and sliced
- 4 cups mixed greens
- 1/2 avocado, sliced
- 1/4 cup cherry tomatoes, halved
- 1/4 cup sliced cucumber
- 2 tbsp olive oil
- 1 tbsp balsamic vinegar
- Salt and pepper to taste

Instructions:

1. Put the cucumber, cherry tomatoes, avocado, and mixed greens in a big bowl.
2. Place sliced steak on top.
3. Drizzle with balsamic vinegar and olive oil.
4. Add salt and pepper to taste, then toss to mix.

Nutritional Values (per serving):

- Calories: 400
- Protein: 28g
- Carbs: 10g
- Fat: 28g
- Fiber: 6g

Health Benefits:

• Rich in good fats and protein.
• Minimal carbohydrates, which promote steady blood sugar levels.
•Vegetables that are fresh offer vital vitamins and antioxidants.

26. Chicken and Cauliflower Tacos

Ingredients:

- 2 cups cauliflower florets
- 1 chicken breast, cooked and shredded

- 1/4 cup diced red onion
- 1/4 cup chopped cilantro
- 1 tbsp lime juice
- 1 tsp cumin
- Salt and pepper to taste
- 4 large lettuce leaves

Instructions:

1. In a food processor, pulse cauliflower florets until they resemble rice.
2. Cook the cauliflower rice in a pan over medium heat until it becomes soft.
3. Combine the cooked cauliflower rice, red onion, cilantro, lime juice, cumin, salt, and pepper in a bowl along with the shredded chicken.
4. Spoon mixture onto leaves of lettuce, then wrap.

Nutritional Values (per serving, 2 tacos):

- Calories: 250
- Protein: 20g
- Carbs: 10g

- Fat: 12g
- Fiber: 6g

Health Benefits:

- High in protein and low in carbs

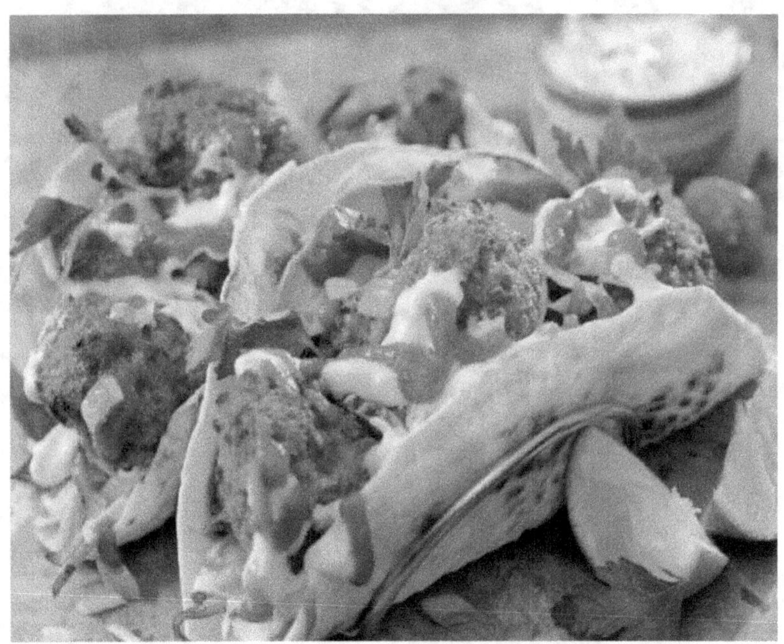

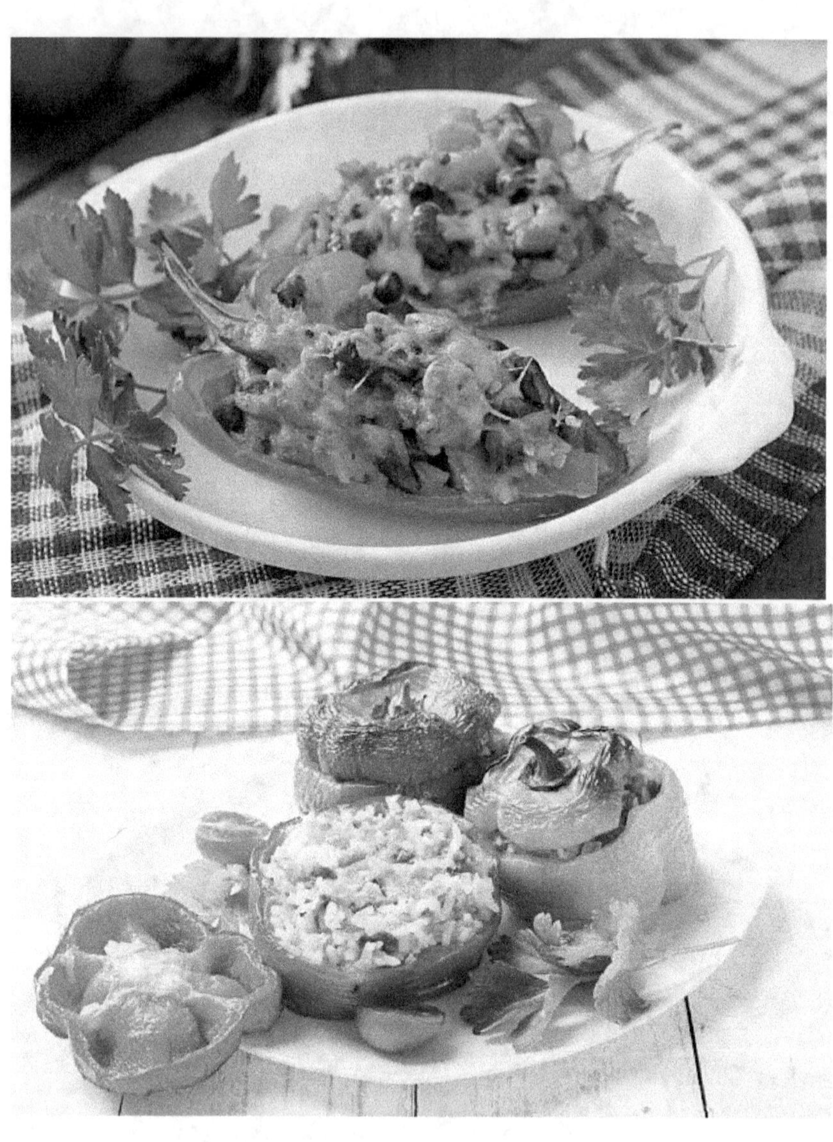

Chapter 3: Dinner Recipes

1. Grilled Salmon with Quinoa Salad

Ingredients:

- 4 salmon fillets
- 1 cup quinoa
- 2 cups water
- 1 cup cherry tomatoes, halved
- 1 cucumber, diced
- 1 red bell pepper, diced
- 1/4 cup red onion, finely chopped
- 2 tbsp olive oil
- 1 lemon, juiced
- Salt and pepper to taste
- Fresh dill for garnish

Instructions:

1. Use cold water to rinse the quinoa. Heat water and quinoa in a saucepan until they boil. After 15

minutes, or until the water is absorbed, reduce heat, cover, and simmer. Use a fork to fluff.

2. Sprinkle salmon fillets with pepper and salt. Cook, turning occasionally, for 4–5 minutes on each side over medium-high heat.

3. Combine the quinoa, cucumber, bell pepper, red onion, and cherry tomatoes in a big bowl.

4. Add a lemon juice and olive oil drizzle. Mix by tossing.

5. Top quinoa salad with salmon fillets and fresh dill for garnish.

Nutritional Values (per serving):

- Calories: 450
- Protein: 35g
- Carbohydrates: 35g
- Fat: 20g
- Fiber: 6g

• Omega-3 fatty acids, which are good for the heart, are abundant in salmon.
• Quinoa helps control blood sugar levels since it is a rich source of protein and fiber.
•Vital vitamins and minerals may be found in vegetables.

2. Chicken and Vegetable Stir-Fry

Ingredients:

- 1 lb boneless, skinless chicken breasts, thinly sliced
- 1 red bell pepper, sliced
- 1 yellow bell pepper, sliced
- 1 cup broccoli florets
- 1 carrot, julienned
- 1 cup snap peas
- 2 garlic cloves, minced
- 1 tbsp ginger, minced
- 2 tbsp low-sodium soy sauce
- 1 tbsp sesame oil

- 1 tbsp olive oil
- 1 tsp cornstarch mixed with 2 tbsp water

Instructions:

1. In a large skillet or wok, heat the olive oil over medium-high heat. When the chicken is no longer pink, add it and simmer.
2. Add the ginger and garlic, and cook for one minute.
3. Include the snap peas, broccoli, carrot, and bell peppers. Sauté the veggies until they are crisp-tender.
4. Add sesame oil and soy sauce and stir. Cook the sauce until it thickens by adding the cornstarch mixture.
5. Present right away.

Nutritional Values (per serving):

- Calories: 320
- Protein: 30g
- Carbohydrates: 15g
- Fat: 15g
- Fiber: 5g

- Lean chicken is a great source of protein.
- Fiber and antioxidants abound in vegetables.
• Low-sodium soy sauce lowers salt consumption, which is good for controlling blood pressure.

3. Turkey and Spinach Stuffed Peppers

Ingredients:

- 4 large bell peppers, tops cut off and seeds removed
- 1 lb ground turkey
- 2 cups fresh spinach, chopped
- 1 cup cooked brown rice
- 1 small onion, diced
- 2 garlic cloves, minced
- 1 tsp dried oregano
- 1 tsp dried basil
- 1/2 cup tomato sauce
- Salt and pepper to taste

- 1/4 cup shredded mozzarella cheese

Instructions:

1. Set oven temperature to 190°C/375°F.
2. Cook the ground turkey, onion, and garlic in a big pan over medium heat until the turkey loses its pink color.
3. Include the cooked brown rice, spinach, basil, oregano, and salt & pepper. Cook until wilted, about 3 minutes.
4. Add tomato sauce and stir.
5. Stuff the turkey mixture into each bell pepper and put them in a baking tray.
6. Place mozzarella shreds on top of every pepper.
7. Bake for twenty-five minutes with a foil cover. After taking off the foil, bake for a further ten minutes to melt the cheese.

Nutritional Values (per serving):

- Calories: 350
- Protein: 25g

- Carbohydrates: 30g
- Fat: 15g
- Fiber: 7g

Health Benefits:

- One source of lean protein is turkey.
- Bell peppers are rich in A and C vitamins.
- Iron and folate are found in spinach.

4. Zucchini Noodles with Pesto and Grilled Chicken

Ingredients:

- 4 zucchinis, spiralized
- 2 boneless, skinless chicken breasts
- 2 cups fresh basil leaves
- 1/4 cup pine nuts
- 1/4 cup Parmesan cheese, grated
- 2 garlic cloves
- 1/4 cup olive oil

- Salt and pepper to taste
- Cherry tomatoes for garnish

Instructions:

1. Sprinkle some salt and pepper on the chicken breasts. Cook for 6–7 minutes on each side on a medium-high grill, or until well done. Cut thinly.
2. Put the garlic, olive oil, Parmesan cheese, pine nuts, and basil leaves in a food processor. Process till smooth.
3. Combine pesto sauce with zucchini noodles.
4. Top the zucchini noodles with cherry tomatoes and chunks of grilled chicken.

Nutritional Values (per serving):

- Calories: 400
- Protein: 35g
- Carbohydrates: 15g
- Fat: 25g
- Fiber: 5g

Health Benefits:

• Noodles of zucchini have a high fiber content and a low carb count.

• Antioxidants and healthy fats are provided by pesto.

• Lean protein sources include grilled chicken.

5. Vegetable and Tofu Stir-Fry

Ingredients:

- 1 block firm tofu, drained and cubed
- 1 cup broccoli florets
- 1 red bell pepper, sliced
- 1 yellow bell pepper, sliced
- 1 cup snap peas
- 1 carrot, julienned
- 2 garlic cloves, minced
- 1 tbsp ginger, minced
- 2 tbsp low-sodium soy sauce
- 1 tbsp sesame oil
- 1 tbsp olive oil

Instructions:

1. In a large skillet or wok, heat the olive oil over medium-high heat. When the tofu is golden brown, add it. Take out and place aside.
2. Sauté the ginger and garlic in the pan for one minute.
3. Include the carrot, snap peas, bell peppers, and broccoli. Sauté the veggies until they are crisp-tender.
4. Add sesame oil and soy sauce and stir. Return the tofu to the skillet and mix everything together.
5. Present right away.

Nutritional Values (per serving):

- Calories: 300
- Protein: 20g
- Carbohydrates: 20g
- Fat: 15g
- Fiber: 5g

- A good source of plant-based protein is tofu.
- Vital vitamins and minerals may be found in vegetables.
- Low-sodium soy sauce aids in reducing salt consumption.

6. Quinoa and Black Bean Stuffed Sweet Potatoes

Ingredients:

- 4 medium sweet potatoes
- 1 cup quinoa
- 2 cups water
- 1 can black beans, rinsed and drained
- 1 cup corn kernels
- 1 red bell pepper, diced
- 1/4 cup red onion, finely chopped
- 1 avocado, diced
- 2 tbsp olive oil
- 1 lime, juiced
- Salt and pepper to taste

- Fresh cilantro for garnish

Instructions:

1. Set oven temperature to 200°C/400°F. Bake sweet potatoes until they are soft, 45 to 50 minutes.
2. Use cool water to rinse the quinoa. Bring water and quinoa to a boil in a saucepan. Once the water has been absorbed, reduce heat, cover, and simmer for fifteen minutes. Using a fork, fluff.
3. Combine the quinoa, black beans, corn, red onion, and bell pepper in a big bowl.
4. Add a lime juice and olive oil drizzle. To mix, toss. Add pepper and salt for seasoning.
5. Cut roasted sweet potatoes in half, then sprinkle quinoa mixture on top.
6. Add avocado and fresh cilantro as garnishes.

Nutritional Values (per serving):

- Calories: 450
- Protein: 15g
- Carbohydrates: 75g

- Fat: 15g
- Fiber: 15g

Health Benefits:

• Vitamins A and C as well as fiber are abundant in sweet potatoes.

• Quinoa and black beans are good sources of fiber and plant-based   protein.

• Avocado contributes good fats.

7. Mediterranean Chickpea Salad

Ingredients:

- 1 can chickpeas, rinsed and drained
- 1 cucumber, diced
- 1 red bell pepper, diced
- 1/2 red onion, finely chopped
- 1/2 cup cherry tomatoes, halved
- 1/4 cup Kalamata olives, sliced
- 1/4 cup feta cheese, crumbled

- 2 tbsp olive oil

- 1 lemon, juiced

- 1 tsp dried oregano

- Salt and pepper to taste

- Fresh parsley for garnish

Instructions:

1. Combine the chickpeas, cucumber, red onion, bell pepper, cherry tomatoes, olives, and feta cheese in a big bowl.

2. Add a lemon juice and olive oil drizzle. Add the pepper, salt, and oregano. To mix, toss.

3. Add fresh parsley as a garnish.

4. Serve right away or store in the fridge for later.

Nutritional Values (per serving):

- Calories: 350

- Protein: 15g

- Carbohydrates: 30g

- Fat: 20g

- Fiber: 10g

- Chickpeas are a good source of protein and fiber.
- Vital vitamins and minerals may be found in vegetables.
- Good fats may be obtained via olives and olive oil.

8. Baked Cod with Lemon and Garlic

Ingredients:

- 4 cod fillets
- 3 garlic cloves, minced
- 1 lemon, thinly sliced
- 2 tbsp olive oil
- Salt and pepper to taste
- Fresh parsley for garnish

Instructions:

1. Set oven temperature to 190°C/375°F.

2. Put the fish fillets on an ovenproof dish. Add a drizzle of olive oil and season with salt, pepper, and garlic.

3. Cover the fish with slices of lemon.

4. Bake for 20 to 25 minutes, or until a fork can easily pierce the fish.

5. Add some fresh parsley as a garnish and serve.

Nutritional Values (per serving):

- Calories: 250
- Protein: 30g
- Carbohydrates: 5g
- Fat: 10g
- Fiber: 1g

Health Benefits:

- One source of lean protein is cod.
- The anti-inflammatory qualities of garlic.
- Vitamin C is present in lemons.

9. Eggplant Parmesan

Ingredients:

- 1 large eggplant, sliced into rounds
- 2 eggs, beaten
- 1 cup whole wheat breadcrumbs
- 1/2 cup grated Parmesan cheese
- 1 cup marinara sauce
- 1 cup shredded mozzarella cheese
- 1 tbsp olive oil
- Fresh basil for garnish

Instructions:

1. Set oven temperature to 190°C/375°F.
2. Coat eggplant slices in a combination of breadcrumbs and Parmesan cheese after dipping them in beaten eggs.
3. In a big skillet over medium heat, preheat the olive oil. Slices of eggplant should be fried till golden brown all over. Transfer to a plate covered with paper towels to drain.

4. Cover a baking dish with a thin coating of marinara sauce. Place the pieces of eggplant on top. Cover the eggplant with the leftover sauce and top with mozzarella cheese.

5. Bake for 20 to 25 minutes, or until bubbling and melted cheese.

6. Add some fresh basil as a garnish and serve.

Nutritional Values (per serving):

- Calories: 350
- Protein: 20g
- Carbohydrates: 30g
- Fat: 15g
- Fiber: 8g

Health Benefits:

- Antioxidants and fiber content are high in eggplant.
- Adding whole wheat breadcrumbs adds more fiber.
- Minerals and vitamins abound in marinara sauce.

10. Lentil and Vegetable Stew

Ingredients:

- 1 cup dried lentils
- 4 cups vegetable broth
- 1 onion, diced
- 2 garlic cloves, minced
- 2 carrots, diced
- 2 celery stalks, diced
- 1 zucchini, diced
- 1 can diced tomatoes
- 1 tsp dried thyme
- 1 tsp dried oregano
- 2 tbsp olive oil
- Salt and pepper to taste

Instructions:

1. In a big saucepan over medium heat, warm the olive oil. Add the garlic and onion and sauté until tender.
2. Include the zucchini, celery, and carrots. Sauté the veggies until they are soft.

3. Add the diced tomatoes, vegetable broth, oregano, thyme, and lentils. Heat till boiling.

4. Lower the heat and cook the lentils for 35 to 40 minutes, or until they become soft.

5. Add pepper and salt for seasoning. Warm up the food.

Nutritional Values (per serving):

- Calories: 300
- Protein: 15g
- Carbohydrates: 45g
- Fat: 8g
- Fiber: 15g

Health Benefits:

• Plant-based fiber and protein may be found in abundance in   lentils.

• Vital vitamins and minerals may be found in vegetables.

• Rich in antioxidants and low in fat.

11. Shrimp and Asparagus Skillet

Ingredients:

- 1 lb shrimp, peeled and deveined
- 1 bunch asparagus, trimmed and cut into pieces
- 2 garlic cloves, minced
- 1 lemon, juiced
- 2 tbsp olive oil
- Salt and pepper to taste
- Fresh parsley for garnish

Instructions:

1. In a large pan over medium-high heat, warm the olive oil. Add the garlic and cook it until aromatic.
2. Add the shrimp and simmer for 3–4 minutes, or until they are pink and opaque.
3. Include asparagus and heat until just crisp-tender.
4. Add a lemon juice drizzle and salt and pepper to taste.
5. Add some fresh parsley as a garnish and serve.

- Calories: 250
- Protein: 25g
- Carbohydrates: 10g
- Fat: 12g
- Fiber: 4g

Health Benefits:

- Shrimp is a high-protein, low-calorie food.
- Asparagus is high in A, C, and K vitamins.
- Its low carb content makes it perfect for controlling blood sugar.

12. Cauliflower Fried Rice

Ingredients:

- 1 head cauliflower, grated into rice-sized pieces
- 2 eggs, beaten
- 1 cup peas and carrots mix

- 1 small onion, diced

- 2 garlic cloves, minced

- 2 tbsp low-sodium soy sauce

- 1 tbsp sesame oil

- 1 tbsp olive oil

- 2 green onions, sliced

Instructions:

1. In a big pan over medium heat, warm the olive oil. Add the garlic and onion and sauté until tender.

2. Cook the carrots and peas until they are soft.

3. Transfer the veggies to the side and cover the pan with the beaten eggs. Cook until thoroughly done.

4. Include the sesame oil, soy sauce, and cauliflower rice. Cook the cauliflower, stirring regularly, until it becomes soft.

5. Add green onions and toss, then serve hot.

Nutritional Values (per serving):

- Calories: 200

- Protein: 10g

- Carbohydrates: 15g
- Fat: 12g
- Fiber: 5g

Health Benefits:

• Carbs are little and cauliflower is strong in fiber.

• Is rich in minerals and vitamins from veggies.

• Using low-sodium soy sauce helps you eat less salt.

13. Grilled Chicken with Avocado Salsa

Ingredients:

- 4 boneless, skinless chicken breasts
- 2 avocados, diced
- 1 tomato, diced
- 1/4 cup red onion, finely chopped
- 1 lime, juiced
- 2 tbsp fresh cilantro, chopped
- 1 tbsp olive oil

- Salt and pepper to taste

Instructions:

1. Sprinkle some salt and pepper on the chicken breasts. Cook for 6–7 minutes on each side on a medium-high grill, or until well done.
2. Add avocados, tomato, red onion, cilantro, lime juice, olive oil, salt, and pepper to a bowl.
3. Present grilled chicken with avocado salsa on top.

Nutritional Values (per serving):

- Calories: 350
- Protein: 30g
- Carbohydrates: 10g
- Fat: 20g
- Fiber: 7g

Health Benefits:

- Lean protein is found in chicken.
- Avocado has a lot of fiber and good fats.
- Onion and tomato provide antioxidants and vitamins.

14. Spaghetti Squash with Turkey Meatballs

Ingredients:

- 1 large spaghetti squash
- 1 lb ground turkey
- 1/2 cup whole wheat breadcrumbs
- 1 egg
- 1/4 cup Parmesan cheese, grated
- 2 garlic cloves, minced
- 1 tsp dried oregano
- 1 tsp dried basil
- 2 cups marinara sauce
- Salt and pepper to taste
- Fresh basil for garnish

Instructions:

1. Set oven temperature to 200°C/400°F. Remove the seeds after cutting the spaghetti squash in half lengthwise. On a baking sheet, place cut-side down,

and bake for 40 to 45 minutes. Use a fork to scrape out the strands.

2. Combine the ground turkey, egg, breadcrumbs, Parmesan cheese, garlic, basil, oregano, and salt and pepper in a bowl. Shape into meatballs.

3. Transfer the meatballs to a baking sheet and simmer for 20 to 25 minutes, or until well cooked.

4. In a saucepan, preheat the marinara sauce over medium heat.

5. Top spaghetti squash with marinara sauce and turkey meatballs. Throw some fresh basil on top.

Nutritional Values (per serving):

- Calories: 400
- Protein: 30g
- Carbohydrates: 30g
- Fat: 15g
- Fiber: 10g

- One form of lean protein is turkey meatballs.
- Squash has a high fiber content and a low carb count.
- Antioxidants and vitamins are added by marinara sauce.

15. Stuffed Portobello Mushrooms

Ingredients:

- 4 large Portobello mushrooms, stems removed
- 1 cup fresh spinach, chopped
- 1/2 cup ricotta cheese
- 1/4 cup Parmesan cheese, grated
- 1 garlic clove, minced
- 1 tbsp olive oil
- Salt and pepper to taste
- Fresh parsley for garnish

Instructions:

1. Set oven temperature to 190°C/375°F.

2. Combine spinach, Parmesan cheese, ricotta cheese, garlic, salt, and pepper in a bowl.

3. Put the mushrooms on a baking pan after brushing them with olive oil.

4. Stuff the spinach mixture into each mushroom.

5. Bake the mushrooms for 20 to 25 minutes, or until they are soft.

6. Add some fresh parsley as a garnish and serve.

Nutritional Values (per serving):

- Calories: 200
- Protein: 10g
- Carbohydrates: 10g
- Fat: 12g
- Fiber: 3g

Health Benefits:

• Portobello mushrooms are packed with of nutrients and low in calories.

• Iron and vitamins are found in spinach.

• Protein and calcium are added via ricotta and parmesan.

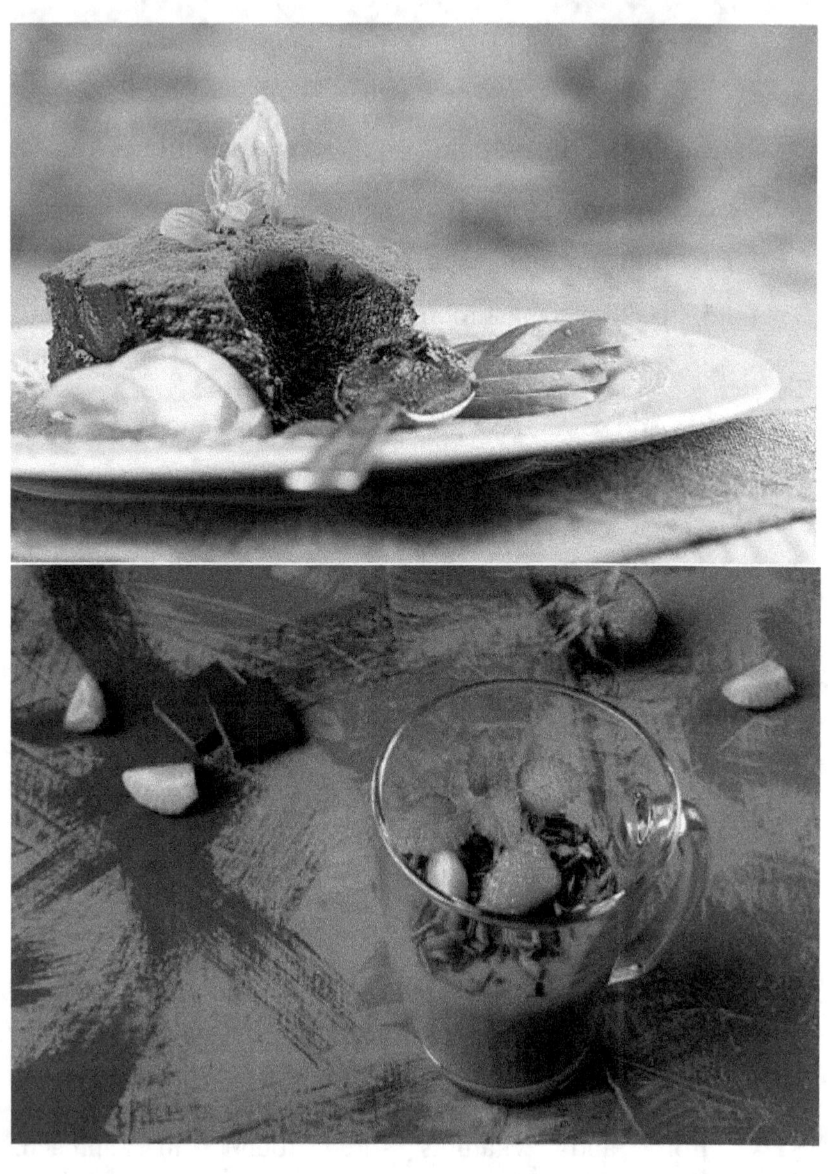

Chapter 4: Desserts

1. Chia Seed Pudding

Ingredients:

- 1/4 cup chia seeds
- 1 cup unsweetened almond milk
- 1 tsp vanilla extract
- 1 tbsp sugar-free sweetener (optional)
- Fresh berries for topping

Instructions:

1. Put the almond milk, sweetener, vanilla extract, and chia seeds in a bowl.
2. Mix thoroughly and leave for ten minutes. Give it another stir to loosen any clumps.
3. For at least four hours or overnight, cover and chill.
4. Garnish with fresh berries and serve.

Nutritional Values (per serving):

- Calories: 120

- Carbohydrates: 12g
- Protein: 4g
- Fat: 7g
- Fiber: 10g

Health Benefits:

• Rich in fiber, which aids with blood sugar regulation.

• Chia seeds' omega-3 fatty acids are good for your heart.

2. Greek Yogurt with Nuts and Berries

Ingredients:

- 1 cup plain Greek yogurt
- 1/4 cup mixed berries (blueberries, strawberries, raspberries)
- 1 tbsp chopped nuts (almonds, walnuts, or pecans)
- 1 tsp honey (optional)

Instructions:

1. Put the Greek yogurt in a dish.
2. Add chopped nuts and mixed berries on top.
3. If desired, drizzle with honey.

Nutritional Values (per serving):

- Calories: 150
- Carbohydrates: 15g
- Protein: 12g
- Fat: 5g
- Fiber: 2g

Health Benefits:

• Packed with protein, which helps you feel fuller for longer.

• Yogurt contains probiotics that promote digestive health.

3. Almond Flour Cookies

Ingredients:

- 1 cup almond flour
- 1/4 cup sugar-free sweetener
- 1/4 tsp baking soda
- 1/4 cup melted coconut oil
- 1 egg
- 1 tsp vanilla extract

Instructions:

1. Set oven temperature to 175°C/350°F.
2. Combine baking soda, sweetener, and almond flour in a bowl.
3. Include the egg, vanilla essence, and heated coconut oil. Stir until well blended.
4. Place dough spoonful onto a parchment paper-lined baking sheet.
5. Bake until the edges are brown, 10 to 12 minutes.

Nutritional Values (per cookie):

- Calories: 100
- Carbohydrates: 2g
- Protein: 3g
- Fat: 9g
- Fiber: 1g

Health Benefits:

• Low in carbohydrates, which means they're good for controlling blood sugar.

• Almond flour offers protein and good fats.

4. Coconut Macaroons

Ingredients:

- 2 cups unsweetened shredded coconut
- 1/2 cup sugar-free sweetener
- 4 egg whites
- 1 tsp vanilla extract

Instructions:

1. Set oven temperature to 325°F, or 165°C.
2. Combine the egg whites, sweetener, shredded coconut, and vanilla extract in a dish.
3. Transfer little mounds onto a parchment paper-lined baking sheet.
4. Bake until golden brown, 20 to 25 minutes.

Nutritional Values (per macaroon):

- Calories: 70
- Carbohydrates: 3g
- Protein: 2g
- Fat: 6g
- Fiber: 2g

Health Benefits:

- Coconut offers fiber and good fats.
- Low in carbohydrates and sugar, making it ideal for managing diabetes.

5. Avocado Chocolate Mousse

Ingredients:

- 2 ripe avocados
- 1/4 cup unsweetened cocoa powder
- 1/4 cup sugar-free sweetener
- 1/4 cup unsweetened almond milk
- 1 tsp vanilla extract

Instructions:

1. Put the avocados, almond milk, sweetener, cocoa powder, and vanilla extract in a blender.
2. Blend until creamy and smooth.
3. Let the food cool in the fridge for a minimum of half an hour before to serving.

Nutritional Values (per serving):

- Calories: 180
- Carbohydrates: 15g
- Protein: 2g

- Fat: 15g
- Fiber: 7g

Health Benefits:

• Avocados are a good source of heart-healthy fats.

• Rich in fiber, which helps regulate blood sugar.

6. Frozen Yogurt Bark

Ingredients:

- 2 cups plain Greek yogurt
- 1/4 cup mixed berries
- 2 tbsp chopped nuts
- 1 tbsp sugar-free sweetener

Instructions:

1. Evenly distribute Greek yogurt onto a parchment paper-lined baking sheet.
2. Add chopped nuts and mixed berries as a sprinkle.
3. If desired, drizzle with sweetness.

4. Freeze until solid, or for at least two hours.

5. Cut into pieces and present.

Nutritional Values (per serving):

- Calories: 90

- Carbohydrates: 9g

- Protein: 8g

- Fat: 3g

- Fiber: 2g

Health Benefits:

- Yogurt's probiotics facilitate digestion.
- Berries are high in fiber and antioxidants.

7. Baked Apple Slices

Ingredients:

- 2 large apples, cored and sliced

- 1 tsp cinnamon

- 1 tbsp sugar-free sweetener
- 1 tbsp lemon juice

Instructions:

1. Set oven temperature to 190°C/375°F.
2. Combine apple slices, sweetener, and lemon juice in a bowl.
3. Arrange apple slices on a parchment paper-lined baking sheet.
4. Bake until soft, 15 to 20 minutes.

Nutritional Values (per serving):

- Calories: 80
- Carbohydrates: 22g
- Protein: 0g
- Fat: 0g
- Fiber: 4g

Health Benefits:

- Rich in fiber, which manages blood sugar levels.
- Vitamins and antioxidants are abundant in apples.

8. Dark Chocolate-Covered Strawberries

Ingredients:

- 1 cup fresh strawberries
- 1/2 cup dark chocolate (70% cocoa or higher), melted

Instructions:

1. Clean and pat strawberries dry.
2. Allow the extra dark chocolate to fall off after dipping each strawberry into the melted chocolate.
3. Transfer to a parchment paper-lined baking sheet.
4. Allow it cool in the fridge until the chocolate solidifies.

Nutritional Values (per serving, 3 strawberries):

- Calories: 100
- Carbohydrates: 15g
- Protein: 1g

- Fat: 6g
- Fiber: 4g

Health Benefits:

- Antioxidants are found in dark chocolate.
- Strawberries provide fiber and vitamins.

9. Pumpkin Spice Muffins

Ingredients:

- 1 cup almond flour
- 1/2 cup pumpkin puree
- 2 eggs
- 1/4 cup sugar-free sweetener
- 1 tsp baking powder
- 1 tsp cinnamon
- 1/2 tsp nutmeg

Instructions:

1. Set oven temperature to 175°C/350°F.

2. Combine almond flour, pureed pumpkin, eggs, sugar, nutmeg, cinnamon, and baking powder in a bowl.

3. Transfer batter into a muffin tray that has paper cups inside.

4. After inserting a toothpick, bake for 20 to 25 minutes, or until it comes out clean.

Nutritional Values (per muffin):

- Calories: 90
- Carbohydrates: 7g
- Protein: 3g
- Fat: 6g
- Fiber: 2g

Health Benefits:

- Rich in fiber and low in carbs.
- Vitamins and antioxidants abound in pumpkin.

10. Blueberry Almond Crumble

Ingredients:

- 2 cups fresh or frozen blueberries
- 1/2 cup almond flour
- 1/4 cup chopped almonds
- 2 tbsp sugar-free sweetener
- 2 tbsp melted coconut oil

Instructions:

1. Set oven temperature to 175°C/350°F.
2. Fill a baking dish with blueberries.
3. Combine melted coconut oil, sweetener, chopped almonds, and almond flour in a bowl.
4. Dredge the blend onto the blueberries.
5. Bake for 20 to 25 minutes, or until brown on top.

Nutritional Values (per serving):

- Calories: 150
- Carbohydrates: 12g

- Protein: 3g

- Fat: 10g

- Fiber: 4g

Health Benefits:

- Blueberries include fiber and antioxidants.
- Almonds provide protein and good fats.

11. Lemon Ricotta Cheesecake

Ingredients:

- 1 cup ricotta cheese
- 1/4 cup sugar-free sweetener
- 2 eggs
- 1 tsp vanilla extract
- Zest and juice of 1 lemon

Instructions:

1. Set oven temperature to 325°F, or 165°C.

2. In a bowl, blend together the ricotta cheese, eggs, sugar, zest, and juice of the lemon until smooth.
3. Transfer mixture to a little baking dish.
4. Bake for 45 to 50 minutes, or until brown and firm.

Nutritional Values (per serving):

- Calories: 120
- Carbohydrates: 5g
- Protein: 9g
- Fat: 7g
- Fiber: 0g

Health Benefits:

- Low carbohydrates and high protein content.
- Vitamin C is found in lemons.

12. Coconut Milk Ice Cream

Ingredients:

- 2 cups full-fat coconut milk

- 1/4 cup sugar-free sweetener
- 1 tsp vanilla extract

Instructions:

1. Combine the sweetener, vanilla extract, and coconut milk in a bowl.
2. Transfer mixture to ice cream machine and churn per manufacturer's directions.
3. Prior to serving, freeze for a minimum of two hours.

Nutritional Values (per serving):

- Calories: 150
- Carbohydrates: 6g
- Protein: 1g
- Fat: 14g
- Fiber: 1g

Health Benefits:

- Low-carb and dairy-free.
- Coconut milk offers good fats.

13. Raspberry Almond Parfait

Ingredients:

- 1 cup plain Greek yogurt
- 1/2 cup fresh raspberries
- 2 tbsp sliced almonds
- 1 tbsp sugar-free sweetener

Instructions:

1. Arrange Greek yogurt, raspberries, and sliced almonds in a dish or glass.
2. If desired, drizzle some sweetness over it.

Nutritional Values (per serving):

- Calories: 160
- Carbohydrates: 15g
- Protein: 12g
- Fat: 7g
- Fiber: 4g

Health Benefits:

- Yogurt's probiotics promote digestive health.
- Fiber and antioxidants are found in raspberries.

14. Chocolate Peanut Butter Fat Bombs

Ingredients:

- 1/2 cup natural peanut butter
- 1/4 cup coconut oil, melted
- 2 tbsp unsweetened cocoa powder
- 2 tbsp sugar-free sweetener

Instructions:

1. Combine peanut butter, sweetener, cocoa powder, and heated coconut oil in a bowl.
2. Transfer mixture to ice cube trays or silicone molds.
3. Before serving, freeze for at least one hour.

Nutritional Values (per serving):

- Calories: 110
- Carbohydrates: 3g
- Protein: 2g
- Fat: 10g
- Fiber: 1g

Health Benefits:

• Rich in good fats, which helps prolong feelings of fullness.

• Low in carbohydrates and good for controlling blood sugar.

15. Banana Oat Cookies

Ingredients:

- 2 ripe bananas, mashed
- 1 cup rolled oats
- 1/4 cup sugar-free chocolate chips (optional)
- 1 tsp cinnamon

Instructions:

1. Set oven temperature to 175°C/350°F.
2. Combine chocolate chips, cinnamon, rolled oats, and mashed bananas in a bowl.
3. Transfer dough by spoonful onto a parchment paper-lined baking sheet.
4. Bake for 15 to 20 minutes, or until fragrant.

Nutritional Values (per cookie):

- Calories: 90
- Carbohydrates: 18g
- Protein: 2g
- Fat: 2g
- Fiber: 2g

Health Benefits:

- Fiber and potassium are found in bananas.
- Soluble fiber, found in oats, aids with blood sugar regulation.

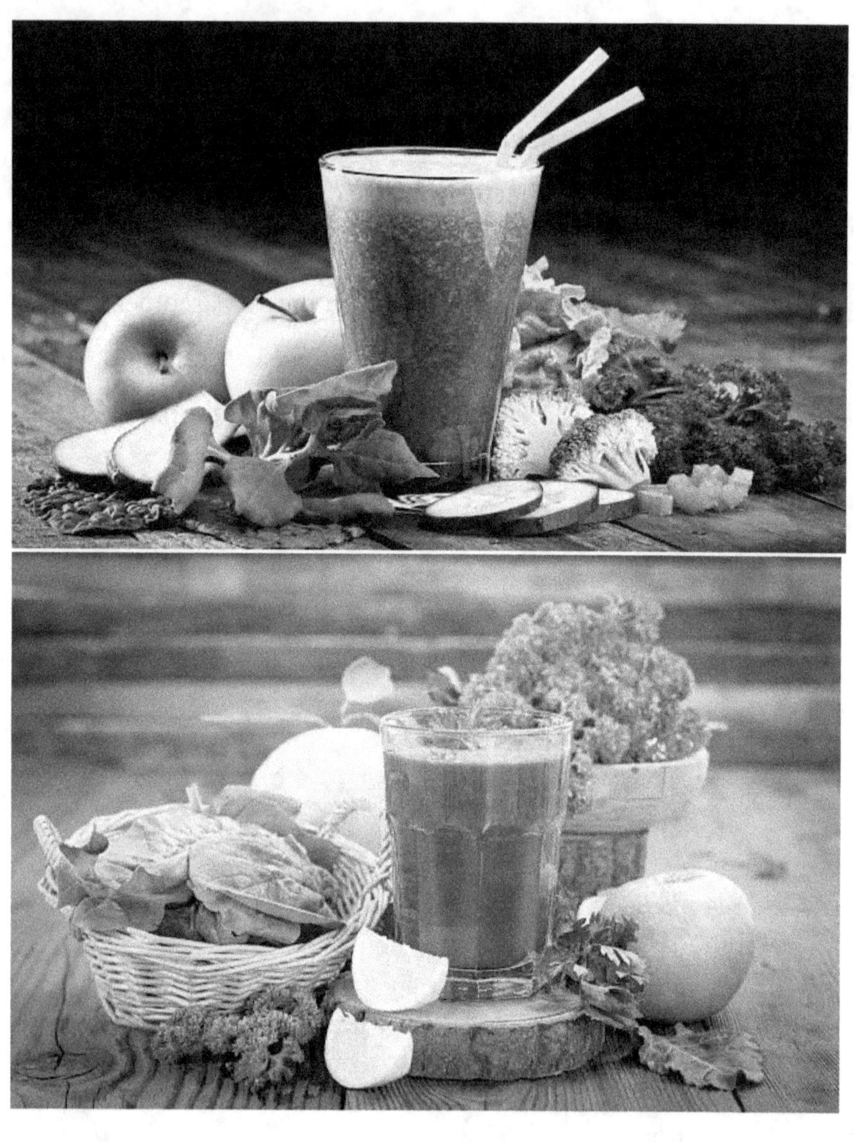

Chapter 5: Beverages

1. Green Smoothie

Ingredients:

- 1 cup unsweetened almond milk
- 1 cup spinach leaves
- 1/2 avocado
- 1/2 green apple
- 1/2 cucumber
- Juice of 1/2 lemon

Instructions:

1. In a blender, combine all ingredients.
2. Blend until uniform.

Nutritional Values (per serving):

- Calories: 150
- Carbohydrates: 15g
- Protein: 3g
- Fat: 10g

- Fiber: 7g

Health Benefits:

• Rich in fiber, which aids with blood sugar regulation.
• Avocado offers good fats.

2. Berry Infused Water

Ingredients:

- 1 cup mixed berries (blueberries, strawberries, raspberries)
- 1 liter water
- Ice cubes

Instructions:

1. Fill a pitcher with water and add berries.
2. Store it in the refrigerator to infuse for at least an hour.
3. Add ice cubes to the dish.

Nutritional Values (per serving):

- Calories: 5
- Carbohydrates: 1g
- Protein: 0g
- Fat: 0g
- Fiber: 0.5g

Health Benefits:

- Low-calorie and hydrating.
- Berries are a good source of antioxidants that promote general health.

3. Iced Herbal Tea

Ingredients:

- 2 herbal tea bags (such as chamomile or peppermint)
- 1liter boiling water
- Ice cubes
- Lemon slices (optional)

Instructions:

1. Boil tea bags in water for five to ten minutes.
2. Take out the tea bags and let the tea settle.
3. Top with ice and, if wanted, garnish with lemon slices.

Nutritional Values (per serving):

- Calories: 0
- Carbohydrates: 0g
- Protein: 0g
- Fat: 0g
- Fiber: 0g

Health Benefits:

- Moisturizing and low in calories.
- Herbal teas can provide a range of calming benefits.

4. Chia Seed Lemonade

Ingredients:

- 2 tbsp chia seeds

- 1 cup water
- Juice of 1 lemon
- 1 tsp sugar-free sweetener

Instructions:

1. Let the chia seeds and water sit for ten minutes.
2. Add the sweetener and lemon juice and stir.

Nutritional Values (per serving):

- Calories: 60
- Carbohydrates: 6g
- Protein: 2g
- Fat: 3g
- Fiber: 5g

Health Benefits:

• Rich in fiber, which helps with blood sugar regulation and digestion.

• Vitamin C is present in lemon juice.

5. Turmeric Latte

Ingredients:

- 1 cup unsweetened almond milk
- 1/2 tsp ground turmeric
- 1/4 tsp ground cinnamon
- 1/4 tsp ground ginger
- 1 tsp sugar-free sweetener

Instructions:

1. Warm up some almond milk in a little pot.
2. Stir in sugar, cinnamon, ginger, and turmeric.
3. Transfer to a cup and serve hot.

Nutritional Values (per serving):

- Calories: 50
- Carbohydrates: 2g
- Protein: 1g
- Fat: 4g
- Fiber: 1g

- Anti-inflammatory qualities are present in turmeric.
- Cinnamon and ginger can aid with blood sugar regulation.

6. Cucumber Mint Cooler

Ingredients:

- 1 cucumber, sliced
- 1/4 cup fresh mint leaves
- 1 liter water
- Ice cubes

Instructions:

1. Fill a pitcher with water and add cucumber slices and mint leaves.
2. Store it in the refrigerator to infuse for at least an hour.
3. Add ice cubes to the dish.

Nutritional Values (per serving):

- Calories: 5

- Carbohydrates: 1g
- Protein: 0g
- Fat: 0g
- Fiber: 0.2g

Health Benefits:

- Refreshing and hydrating.
- Digestion is aided by mint.

7. Cinnamon Spiced Coffee

Ingredients:

- 1 cup brewed coffee
- 1/4 tsp ground cinnamon
- 1 tsp sugar-free sweetener
- 1/4 cup unsweetened almond milk

1.   Prepared   coffee   as   normal.
2.   Stir   in   sugar   and   ground   cinnamon.
3. Thoroughly combine with almond milk.

Nutritional Values (per serving):

- Calories: 30
- Carbohydrates: 2g
- Protein: 1g
- Fat: 2g
- Fiber: 0.5g

Health Benefits:

- Cinnamon can aid with blood sugar regulation.
- Minimal in fat and calories.

8. Green Tea with Lemon

Ingredients:

- 1 green tea bag

- 1 cup boiling water
- Juice of 1/2 lemon

Instructions:

1. Boil a green tea bag for three to five minutes.
2. Remove the tea bag and squeeze in the lemon.
3. Place on ice or serve warm.

Nutritional Values (per serving):

- Calories: 5
- Carbohydrates: 1g
- Protein: 0g
- Fat: 0g
- Fiber: 0g

Health Benefits:

- Antioxidants are present in green tea.
- Vitamin C is added via lemon juice.

9. Berry Smoothie

Ingredients:

- 1 cup unsweetened almond milk
- 1/2 cup mixed berries (blueberries, strawberries, raspberries)
- 1/4 cup plain Greek yogurt
- 1 tsp chia seeds

Instructions:

1. Blend together all of the ingredients.
2. Mix until well combined.

Nutritional Values (per serving):

- Calories: 120
- Carbohydrates: 15g
- Protein: 5g
- Fat: 5g
- Fiber: 4g

Health Benefits:

- Berries are high in fiber and antioxidants.
- Greek yogurt enhances probiotics and protein.

10. Coconut Water with Lime

Ingredients:

- 1 cup coconut water
- Juice of 1 lime
- Ice cubes

Instructions:

1. Combine the lime juice and coconut water.
2. Place on top of ice cubes.

Nutritional Values (per serving):

- Calories: 45
- Carbohydrates: 10g
- Protein: 0g
- Fat: 0g
- Fiber: 1g

Health Benefits:

- Low-calorie and hydrating.
- Electrolytes are provided by coconut water.

11. Protein Shake

Ingredients:

- 1 cup unsweetened almond milk
- 1 scoop sugar-free protein powder
- 1/2 banana
- 1 tsp flaxseeds

Instructions:

1. Fill a blender with all the ingredients.
2. Purée until silky.

Nutritional Values (per serving):

- Calories: 150
- Carbohydrates: 15g
- Protein: 20g

- Fat: 5g
- Fiber: 4g

Health Benefits:

• Rich in protein, which helps to maintain muscular mass.

•Flaxseeds are a good source of fiber and omega-3 fatty acids.

12. Carrot Ginger Juice

Ingredients:

- 2 large carrots
- 1-inch piece of fresh ginger
- 1 apple
- 1/2 lemon

Instructions:

1. Use a juicer to juice the carrots, ginger, apple, and lemon.
2. Mix well, then serve.

- Calories: 90

- Carbohydrates: 22g

- Protein: 1g

- Fat: 0g

- Fiber: 2g

Health Benefits:

• Antioxidants and beta-carotene are found in carrots.

• Ginger possesses anti-inflammatory and digestion-promoting qualities.

13. Spiced Almond Milk

Ingredients:

- 1 cup unsweetened almond milk

- 1/4 tsp ground cinnamon

- 1/4 tsp ground nutmeg

- 1 tsp sugar-free sweetener

Instructions:

1. Warm up some almond milk in a little pot.
2. Stir in sugar, nutmeg, and cinnamon.
3. Transfer to a cup and serve hot.

Nutritional Values (per serving):

- Calories: 40
- Carbohydrates: 2g
- Protein: 1g
- Fat: 3g
- Fiber: 1g

Health Benefits:

• Nutmeg and cinnamon are among the spices that can help control blood sugar.
• Minimal in fat and calories.

14. Tomato Juice with Basil

Ingredients:

- 1 cup tomato juice (low-sodium)

- 1 tbsp fresh basil, chopped
- Dash of black pepper

Instructions:

1. In a glass, mix tomato juice, chopped basil, and black pepper.
2. If desired, pour over ice and stir thoroughly.

Nutritional Values (per serving):

- Calories: 30
- Carbohydrates: 7g
- Protein: 1g
- Fat: 0g
- Fiber: 1g

Health Benefits:

- Antioxidants and vitamins may be found in tomatoes.
- Basil has the ability to reduce inflammation.

15. Vanilla Almond Smoothie

Ingredients:

- 1 cup unsweetened almond milk
- 1/4 cup plain Greek yogurt
- 1/2 tsp vanilla extract
- 1 tbsp almond butter
- 1 tsp sugar-free sweetener

Instructions:

1. Fill a blender with all the ingredients.
2. Purée until silky.

Nutritional Values (per serving):

- Calories: 160
- Carbohydrates: 8g
- Protein: 8g
- Fat: 11g
- Fiber: 2g

- Almond butter offers protein and good fats.
- Greek yogurt increases protein and probiotics.

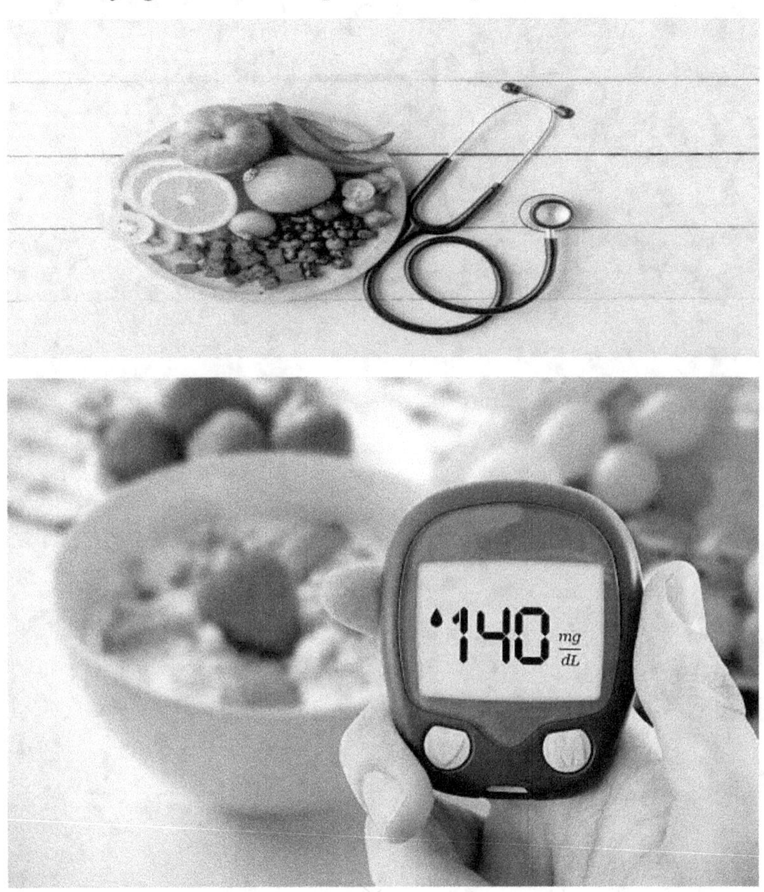

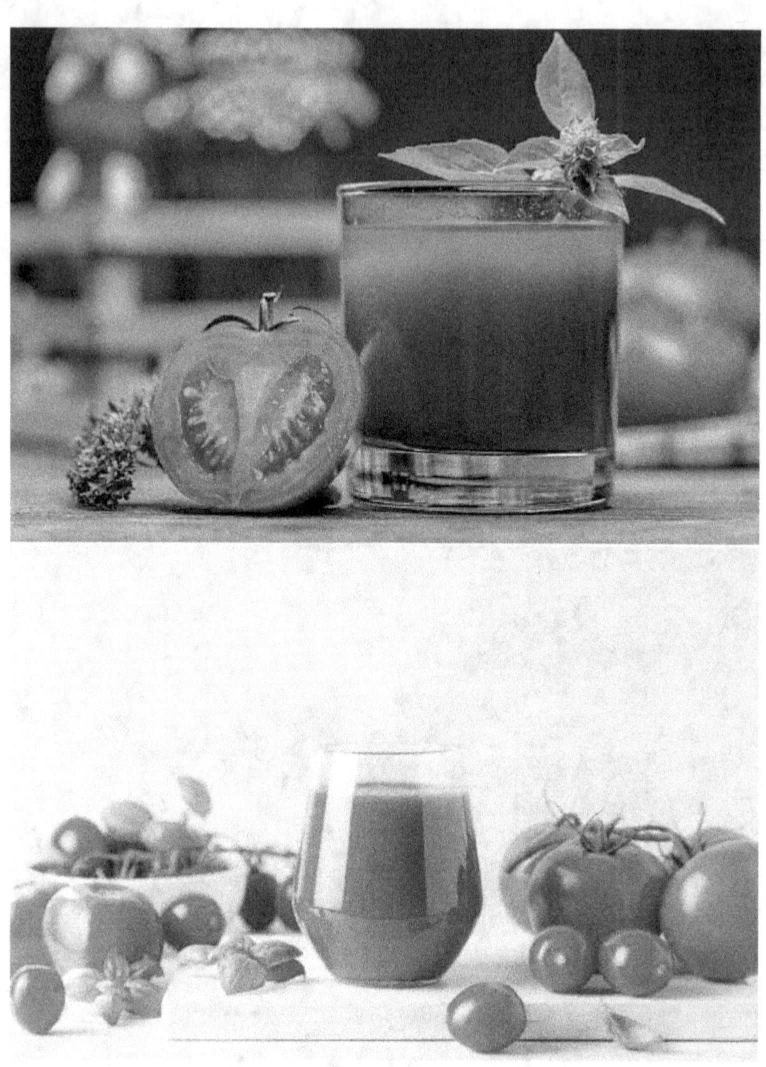

Chapter 6: Additional Resources

Accepting a Healthier Life: Our Type 2 Diabetes Cookbook's Core

Living with Type 2 diabetes is a journey that affects all part of your life; it's more than just managing a medical condition. It might seem like an uphill struggle, from the first shock of the diagnosis to the continual difficulty of juggling medicine, exercise, and food. But this cookbook is meant to serve as a reminder that you are not alone. We hope that every page will help, encourage, and inspire you to take back control of your health and rediscover the pleasure of eating.

A   Transformative   Journey

When Type 2 diabetes is diagnosed, a person may experience a range of feelings, including anxiety, bewilderment, and perhaps a sense of loss. The idea of altering ingrained dietary patterns might be intimidating. However, think of this book as a travel companion for a happier, healthier existence. Considering the emotional difficulties associated with managing diabetes, every meal and piece of advice has been thoughtfully and compassionately created.

Eating as a Feeling Experience

Food serves as much more than just nourishment; it also fosters pleasure, comfort, and cultural ties. It might seem like someone is taking away your identity when you're urged to change your diet. This cookbook aims to demonstrate that you don't have to give up your favorite meals in order to adjust to a diabetic-friendly diet. Rather, the fun part is finding new and interesting ways to enjoy them.

Every dish in this book is designed to be both tasty and healthful, ranging from classic comfort meals to brand-new culinary explorations. Our goal is for your meals to be something you look forward to rather than something you merely have to eat.

Understanding as Strengthening

Understanding how various meals impact your blood sugar levels is essential to managing Type 2 diabetes. This cookbook is more than simply a list of recipes; it's a thorough reference that gives you the information you need to make wise decisions. You will discover the meaning of the glycemic index, the benefits of fiber, the function of protein, and the way to include good fats in your diet. Equipped with this understanding, you may approach your meals with self-assurance and inventiveness.

Narratives of Hope and Adaptability

You will come across first-person accounts in the book from folks who have gone through similar struggles as you. These personal accounts provide encouragement and useful advice, demonstrating that Type 2 diabetes can be managed while still leading a full and fulfilling life. These tales demonstrate the resiliency of the human spirit and the influence of a strong sense of community.

Honoring Food and Health

This cookbook is ultimately a celebration of life, health, and food. It's about appreciating the vivid flavors and textures of healthful foods and finding happiness in providing your body with nourishment. The recipes emphasize whole ingredients and balanced nutrition, and they are meant to be easy to make yet still very tasty.

Establishing Relationships

Making and sharing food with people is a great way to build relationships. You are encouraged to include your friends and family in your journey by this book. You may foster a welcoming environment where others appreciate and comprehend your dietary requirements by sharing these dishes. Food has the power to unite us and, when prepared correctly, to improve our health.

How to Get Well in the Future

This cookbook is a lifeline for those with Type 2 diabetes, not merely a reference. It is here to guide you with elegance and simplicity through the intricacies of managing your diabetes. Every dish is a step toward a better you, a future you own and are proud of. Take a bite, taste something new, and rediscover the pleasure of eating. We are privileged to be a part of your path toward improved health, which begins here.

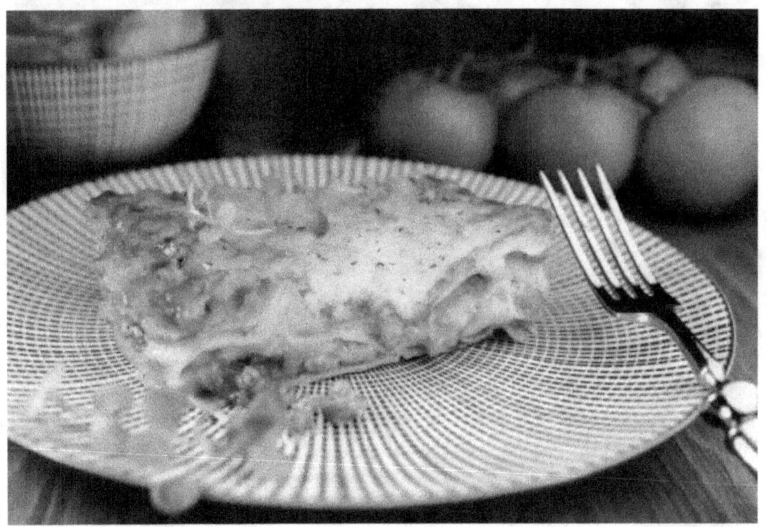

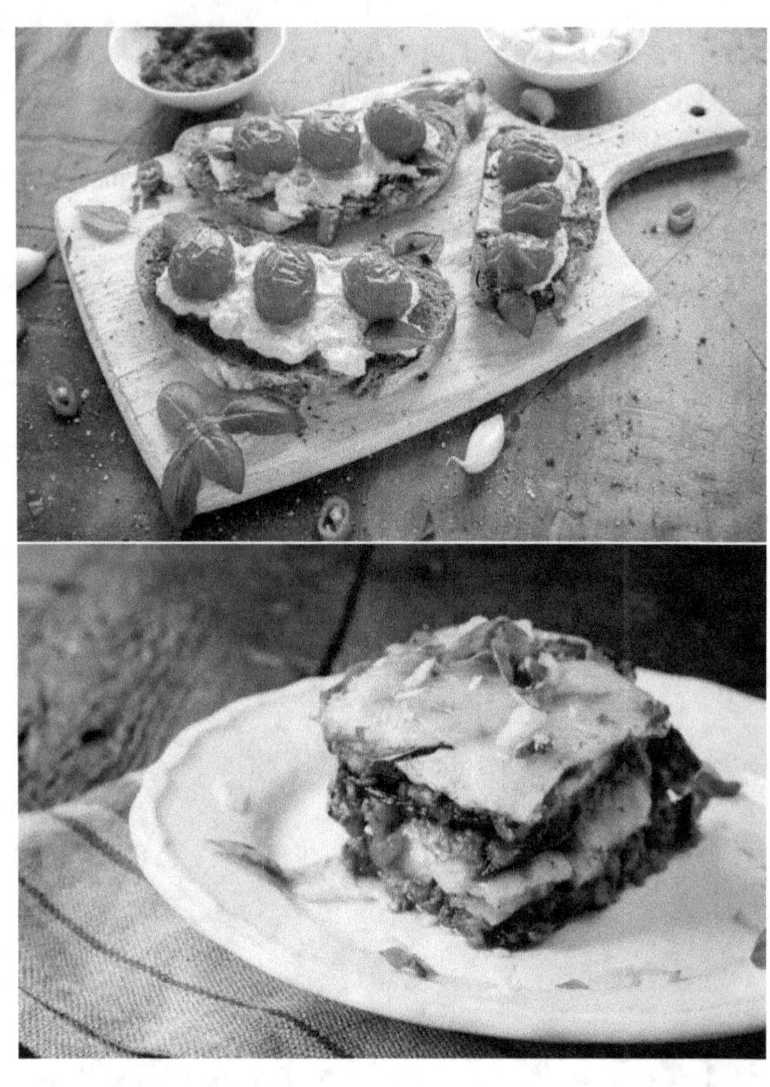

Chapter 7: Bonuses

Weekly Meal planner...(30 pages)

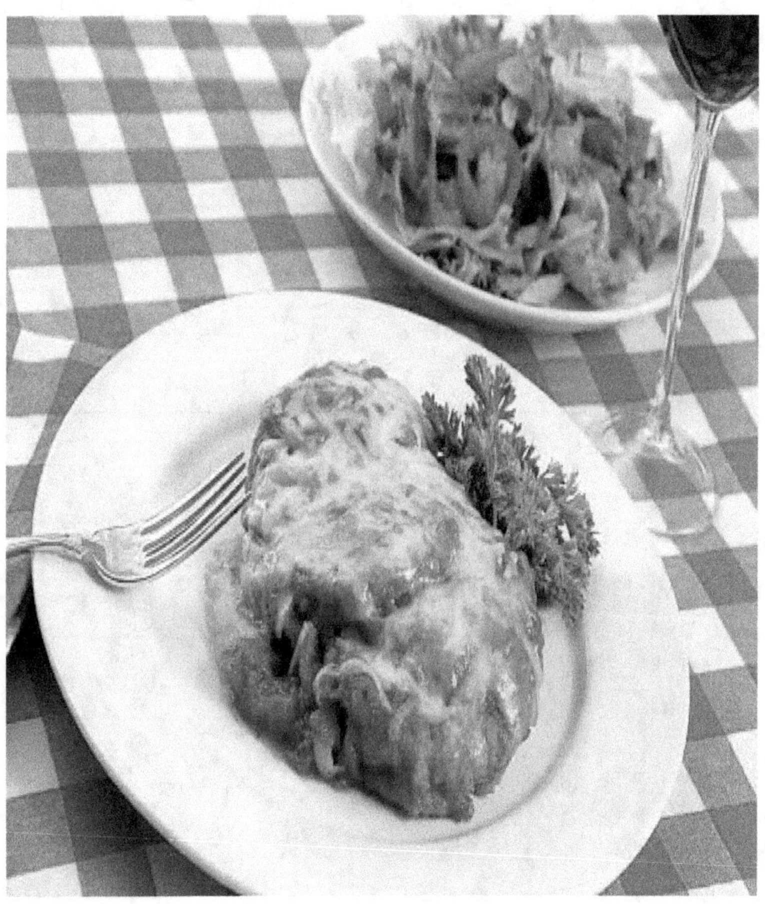

WEEKLY MEAL PLANNER

DATE:

MONDAY

BREAKFAST ___________________

LUNCH___________________

SNACKS ___________________

DINNER___________________

TUESDAY

BREAKFAST ___________________

LUNCH___________________

SNACKS ___________________

DINNER___________________

WEDNESDAY

BREAKFAST ___________________

LUNCH___________________

SNACKS ___________________

DINNER___________________

THURSDAY

BREAKFAST ___________________

LUNCH___________________

SNACKS ___________________

DINNER___________________

FRIDAY

BREAKFAST ___________________

LUNCH___________________

SNACKS ___________________

DINNER___________________

SATURDAY

BREAKFAST ___________________

LUNCH___________________

SNACKS ___________________

DINNER___________________

SUNDAY

BREAKFAST ___________________

LUNCH___________________

SNACKS ___________________

DINNER___________________

NOTES

____

____

____

____

WEEKLY MEAL PLANNER

DATE:

MONDAY

BREAKFAST ______________________

LUNCH ______________________

SNACKS ______________________

DINNER ______________________

TUESDAY

BREAKFAST ______________________

LUNCH ______________________

SNACKS ______________________

DINNER ______________________

WEDNESDAY

BREAKFAST ______________________

LUNCH ______________________

SNACKS ______________________

DINNER ______________________

THURSDAY

BREAKFAST ______________________

LUNCH ______________________

SNACKS ______________________

DINNER ______________________

FRIDAY

BREAKFAST ______________________

LUNCH ______________________

SNACKS ______________________

DINNER ______________________

SATURDAY

BREAKFAST ______________________

LUNCH ______________________

SNACKS ______________________

DINNER ______________________

SUNDAY

BREAKFAST ______________________

LUNCH ______________________

SNACKS ______________________

DINNER ______________________

NOTES

____

____

____

____

WEEKLY MEAL PLANNER

DATE:

MONDAY

BREAKFAST ___________________

LUNCH ___________________

SNACKS ___________________

DINNER ___________________

TUESDAY

BREAKFAST ___________________

LUNCH ___________________

SNACKS ___________________

DINNER ___________________

WEDNESDAY

BREAKFAST ___________________

LUNCH ___________________

SNACKS ___________________

DINNER ___________________

THURSDAY

BREAKFAST ___________________

LUNCH ___________________

SNACKS ___________________

DINNER ___________________

FRIDAY

BREAKFAST ___________________

LUNCH ___________________

SNACKS ___________________

DINNER ___________________

SATURDAY

BREAKFAST ___________________

LUNCH ___________________

SNACKS ___________________

DINNER ___________________

SUNDAY

BREAKFAST ___________________

LUNCH ___________________

SNACKS ___________________

DINNER ___________________

NOTES

____

____

____

____

WEEKLY MEAL PLANNER

DATE:

MONDAY

BREAKFAST _______________

LUNCH _______________

SNACKS _______________

DINNER _______________

TUESDAY

BREAKFAST _______________

LUNCH _______________

SNACKS _______________

DINNER _______________

WEDNESDAY

BREAKFAST _______________

LUNCH _______________

SNACKS _______________

DINNER _______________

THURSDAY

BREAKFAST _______________

LUNCH _______________

SNACKS _______________

DINNER _______________

FRIDAY

BREAKFAST _______________

LUNCH _______________

SNACKS _______________

DINNER _______________

SATURDAY

BREAKFAST _______________

LUNCH _______________

SNACKS _______________

DINNER _______________

SUNDAY

BREAKFAST _______________

LUNCH _______________

SNACKS _______________

DINNER _______________

NOTES

____

____

____

____

WEEKLY MEAL PLANNER

DATE:

MONDAY

BREAKFAST _______________

LUNCH _______________

SNACKS _______________

DINNER _______________

TUESDAY

BREAKFAST _______________

LUNCH _______________

SNACKS _______________

DINNER _______________

WEDNESDAY

BREAKFAST _______________

LUNCH _______________

SNACKS _______________

DINNER _______________

THURSDAY

BREAKFAST _______________

LUNCH _______________

SNACKS _______________

DINNER _______________

FRIDAY

BREAKFAST _______________

LUNCH _______________

SNACKS _______________

DINNER _______________

SATURDAY

BREAKFAST _______________

LUNCH _______________

SNACKS _______________

DINNER _______________

SUNDAY

BREAKFAST _______________

LUNCH _______________

SNACKS _______________

DINNER _______________

NOTES

____

____

____

____

WEEKLY MEAL PLANNER

DATE:

MONDAY

BREAKFAST _______________________

LUNCH _______________________

SNACKS _______________________

DINNER _______________________

TUESDAY

BREAKFAST _______________________

LUNCH _______________________

SNACKS _______________________

DINNER _______________________

WEDNESDAY

BREAKFAST _______________________

LUNCH _______________________

SNACKS _______________________

DINNER _______________________

THURSDAY

BREAKFAST _______________________

LUNCH _______________________

SNACKS _______________________

DINNER _______________________

FRIDAY

BREAKFAST _______________________

LUNCH _______________________

SNACKS _______________________

DINNER _______________________

SATURDAY

BREAKFAST _______________________

LUNCH _______________________

SNACKS _______________________

DINNER _______________________

SUNDAY

BREAKFAST _______________________

LUNCH _______________________

SNACKS _______________________

DINNER _______________________

NOTES

____

____

____

____

WEEKLY MEAL PLANNER

DATE:

MONDAY

BREAKFAST ___________________

LUNCH ___________________

SNACKS ___________________

DINNER ___________________

TUESDAY

BREAKFAST ___________________

LUNCH ___________________

SNACKS ___________________

DINNER ___________________

WEDNESDAY

BREAKFAST ___________________

LUNCH ___________________

SNACKS ___________________

DINNER ___________________

THURSDAY

BREAKFAST ___________________

LUNCH ___________________

SNACKS ___________________

DINNER ___________________

FRIDAY

BREAKFAST ___________________

LUNCH ___________________

SNACKS ___________________

DINNER ___________________

SATURDAY

BREAKFAST ___________________

LUNCH ___________________

SNACKS ___________________

DINNER ___________________

SUNDAY

BREAKFAST ___________________

LUNCH ___________________

SNACKS ___________________

DINNER ___________________

NOTES

____

____

____

____

WEEKLY MEAL PLANNER

DATE:

BREAKFAST _______________________

LUNCH _______________________

SNACKS _______________________

DINNER _______________________

BREAKFAST _______________________

LUNCH _______________________

SNACKS _______________________

DINNER _______________________

BREAKFAST _______________________

LUNCH _______________________

SNACKS _______________________

DINNER _______________________

BREAKFAST _______________________

LUNCH _______________________

SNACKS _______________________

DINNER _______________________

BREAKFAST _______________________

LUNCH _______________________

SNACKS _______________________

DINNER _______________________

BREAKFAST _______________________

LUNCH _______________________

SNACKS _______________________

DINNER _______________________

BREAKFAST _______________________

LUNCH _______________________

SNACKS _______________________

DINNER _______________________

____

____

____

____

WEEKLY MEAL PLANNER

DATE:

MONDAY

BREAKFAST ___________________

LUNCH ___________________

SNACKS ___________________

DINNER ___________________

TUESDAY

BREAKFAST ___________________

LUNCH ___________________

SNACKS ___________________

DINNER ___________________

WEDNESDAY

BREAKFAST ___________________

LUNCH ___________________

SNACKS ___________________

DINNER ___________________

THURSDAY

BREAKFAST ___________________

LUNCH ___________________

SNACKS ___________________

DINNER ___________________

FRIDAY

BREAKFAST ___________________

LUNCH ___________________

SNACKS ___________________

DINNER ___________________

SATURDAY

BREAKFAST ___________________

LUNCH ___________________

SNACKS ___________________

DINNER ___________________

SUNDAY

BREAKFAST ___________________

LUNCH ___________________

SNACKS ___________________

DINNER ___________________

NOTES

____

____

____

____

WEEKLY MEAL PLANNER   DATE:

MONDAY

BREAKFAST ______________________

LUNCH ______________________

SNACKS ______________________

DINNER ______________________

TUESDAY

BREAKFAST ______________________

LUNCH ______________________

SNACKS ______________________

DINNER ______________________

WEDNESDAY

BREAKFAST ______________________

LUNCH ______________________

SNACKS ______________________

DINNER ______________________

THURSDAY

BREAKFAST ______________________

LUNCH ______________________

SNACKS ______________________

DINNER ______________________

FRIDAY

BREAKFAST ______________________

LUNCH ______________________

SNACKS ______________________

DINNER ______________________

SATURDAY

BREAKFAST ______________________

LUNCH ______________________

SNACKS ______________________

DINNER ______________________

SUNDAY

BREAKFAST ______________________

LUNCH ______________________

SNACKS ______________________

DINNER ______________________

NOTES

____

____

____

____

WEEKLY MEAL PLANNER

DATE:

MONDAY

BREAKFAST __________________

LUNCH __________________

SNACKS __________________

DINNER __________________

TUESDAY

BREAKFAST __________________

LUNCH __________________

SNACKS __________________

DINNER __________________

WEDNESDAY

BREAKFAST __________________

LUNCH __________________

SNACKS __________________

DINNER __________________

THURSDAY

BREAKFAST __________________

LUNCH __________________

SNACKS __________________

DINNER __________________

FRIDAY

BREAKFAST __________________

LUNCH __________________

SNACKS __________________

DINNER __________________

SATURDAY

BREAKFAST __________________

LUNCH __________________

SNACKS __________________

DINNER __________________

SUNDAY

BREAKFAST __________________

LUNCH __________________

SNACKS __________________

DINNER __________________

NOTES

____

____

____

____

WEEKLY MEAL PLANNER

DATE:

MONDAY

BREAKFAST ___________________

LUNCH ___________________

SNACKS ___________________

DINNER ___________________

TUESDAY

BREAKFAST ___________________

LUNCH ___________________

SNACKS ___________________

DINNER ___________________

WEDNESDAY

BREAKFAST ___________________

LUNCH ___________________

SNACKS ___________________

DINNER ___________________

THURSDAY

BREAKFAST ___________________

LUNCH ___________________

SNACKS ___________________

DINNER ___________________

FRIDAY

BREAKFAST ___________________

LUNCH ___________________

SNACKS ___________________

DINNER ___________________

SATURDAY

BREAKFAST ___________________

LUNCH ___________________

SNACKS ___________________

DINNER ___________________

SUNDAY

BREAKFAST ___________________

LUNCH ___________________

SNACKS ___________________

DINNER ___________________

NOTES

____

____

____

____

WEEKLY MEAL PLANNER

DATE:

MONDAY

BREAKFAST _______________

LUNCH _______________

SNACKS _______________

DINNER _______________

TUESDAY

BREAKFAST _______________

LUNCH _______________

SNACKS _______________

DINNER _______________

WEDNESDAY

BREAKFAST _______________

LUNCH _______________

SNACKS _______________

DINNER _______________

THURSDAY

BREAKFAST _______________

LUNCH _______________

SNACKS _______________

DINNER _______________

FRIDAY

BREAKFAST _______________

LUNCH _______________

SNACKS _______________

DINNER _______________

SATURDAY

BREAKFAST _______________

LUNCH _______________

SNACKS _______________

DINNER _______________

SUNDAY

BREAKFAST _______________

LUNCH _______________

SNACKS _______________

DINNER _______________

NOTES

____

____

____

____

WEEKLY MEAL PLANNER

DATE:

MONDAY

BREAKFAST ___________________

LUNCH ___________________

SNACKS ___________________

DINNER ___________________

TUESDAY

BREAKFAST ___________________

LUNCH ___________________

SNACKS ___________________

DINNER ___________________

WEDNESDAY

BREAKFAST ___________________

LUNCH ___________________

SNACKS ___________________

DINNER ___________________

THURSDAY

BREAKFAST ___________________

LUNCH ___________________

SNACKS ___________________

DINNER ___________________

FRIDAY

BREAKFAST ___________________

LUNCH ___________________

SNACKS ___________________

DINNER ___________________

SATURDAY

BREAKFAST ___________________

LUNCH ___________________

SNACKS ___________________

DINNER ___________________

SUNDAY

BREAKFAST ___________________

LUNCH ___________________

SNACKS ___________________

DINNER ___________________

NOTES

____

____

____

____

WEEKLY MEAL PLANNER

DATE:

MONDAY

BREAKFAST _______________

LUNCH _______________

SNACKS _______________

DINNER _______________

TUESDAY

BREAKFAST _______________

LUNCH _______________

SNACKS _______________

DINNER _______________

WEDNESDAY

BREAKFAST _______________

LUNCH _______________

SNACKS _______________

DINNER _______________

THURSDAY

BREAKFAST _______________

LUNCH _______________

SNACKS _______________

DINNER _______________

FRIDAY

BREAKFAST _______________

LUNCH _______________

SNACKS _______________

DINNER _______________

SATURDAY

BREAKFAST _______________

LUNCH _______________

SNACKS _______________

DINNER _______________

SUNDAY

BREAKFAST _______________

LUNCH _______________

SNACKS _______________

DINNER _______________

NOTES

____

____

____

____

WEEKLY MEAL PLANNER

DATE:

MONDAY

BREAKFAST _______________

LUNCH _______________

SNACKS _______________

DINNER _______________

TUESDAY

BREAKFAST _______________

LUNCH _______________

SNACKS _______________

DINNER _______________

WEDNESDAY

BREAKFAST _______________

LUNCH _______________

SNACKS _______________

DINNER _______________

THURSDAY

BREAKFAST _______________

LUNCH _______________

SNACKS _______________

DINNER _______________

FRIDAY

BREAKFAST _______________

LUNCH _______________

SNACKS _______________

DINNER _______________

SATURDAY

BREAKFAST _______________

LUNCH _______________

SNACKS _______________

DINNER _______________

SUNDAY

BREAKFAST _______________

LUNCH _______________

SNACKS _______________

DINNER _______________

NOTES

____

____

____

____

WEEKLY MEAL PLANNER

DATE:

MONDAY

BREAKFAST ___________________

LUNCH ___________________

SNACKS ___________________

DINNER ___________________

TUESDAY

BREAKFAST ___________________

LUNCH ___________________

SNACKS ___________________

DINNER ___________________

WEDNESDAY

BREAKFAST ___________________

LUNCH ___________________

SNACKS ___________________

DINNER ___________________

THURSDAY

BREAKFAST ___________________

LUNCH ___________________

SNACKS ___________________

DINNER ___________________

FRIDAY

BREAKFAST ___________________

LUNCH ___________________

SNACKS ___________________

DINNER ___________________

SATURDAY

BREAKFAST ___________________

LUNCH ___________________

SNACKS ___________________

DINNER ___________________

SUNDAY

BREAKFAST ___________________

LUNCH ___________________

SNACKS ___________________

DINNER ___________________

NOTES

____

____

____

____

WEEKLY MEAL PLANNER

DATE:

MONDAY

BREAKFAST __________________

LUNCH __________________

SNACKS __________________

DINNER __________________

TUESDAY

BREAKFAST __________________

LUNCH __________________

SNACKS __________________

DINNER __________________

WEDNESDAY

BREAKFAST __________________

LUNCH __________________

SNACKS __________________

DINNER __________________

THURSDAY

BREAKFAST __________________

LUNCH __________________

SNACKS __________________

DINNER __________________

FRIDAY

BREAKFAST __________________

LUNCH __________________

SNACKS __________________

DINNER __________________

SATURDAY

BREAKFAST __________________

LUNCH __________________

SNACKS __________________

DINNER __________________

SUNDAY

BREAKFAST __________________

LUNCH __________________

SNACKS __________________

DINNER __________________

NOTES

____

____

____

____

WEEKLY MEAL PLANNER

DATE:

MONDAY

BREAKFAST ___________________

LUNCH ___________________

SNACKS ___________________

DINNER ___________________

TUESDAY

BREAKFAST ___________________

LUNCH ___________________

SNACKS ___________________

DINNER ___________________

WEDNESDAY

BREAKFAST ___________________

LUNCH ___________________

SNACKS ___________________

DINNER ___________________

THURSDAY

BREAKFAST ___________________

LUNCH ___________________

SNACKS ___________________

DINNER ___________________

FRIDAY

BREAKFAST ___________________

LUNCH ___________________

SNACKS ___________________

DINNER ___________________

SATURDAY

BREAKFAST ___________________

LUNCH ___________________

SNACKS ___________________

DINNER ___________________

SUNDAY

BREAKFAST ___________________

LUNCH ___________________

SNACKS ___________________

DINNER ___________________

NOTES

____

____

____

____

WEEKLY MEAL PLANNER

DATE:

MONDAY

BREAKFAST _______________

LUNCH _______________

SNACKS _______________

DINNER _______________

TUESDAY

BREAKFAST _______________

LUNCH _______________

SNACKS _______________

DINNER _______________

WEDNESDAY

BREAKFAST _______________

LUNCH _______________

SNACKS _______________

DINNER _______________

THURSDAY

BREAKFAST _______________

LUNCH _______________

SNACKS _______________

DINNER _______________

FRIDAY

BREAKFAST _______________

LUNCH _______________

SNACKS _______________

DINNER _______________

SATURDAY

BREAKFAST _______________

LUNCH _______________

SNACKS _______________

DINNER _______________

SUNDAY

BREAKFAST _______________

LUNCH _______________

SNACKS _______________

DINNER _______________

NOTES

____

____

____

____

WEEKLY MEAL PLANNER

DATE:

MONDAY

BREAKFAST ___________________

LUNCH ___________________

SNACKS ___________________

DINNER ___________________

TUESDAY

BREAKFAST ___________________

LUNCH ___________________

SNACKS ___________________

DINNER ___________________

WEDNESDAY

BREAKFAST ___________________

LUNCH ___________________

SNACKS ___________________

DINNER ___________________

THURSDAY

BREAKFAST ___________________

LUNCH ___________________

SNACKS ___________________

DINNER ___________________

FRIDAY

BREAKFAST ___________________

LUNCH ___________________

SNACKS ___________________

DINNER ___________________

SATURDAY

BREAKFAST ___________________

LUNCH ___________________

SNACKS ___________________

DINNER ___________________

SUNDAY

BREAKFAST ___________________

LUNCH ___________________

SNACKS ___________________

DINNER ___________________

NOTES

____

____

____

____

WEEKLY MEAL PLANNER

DATE:

MONDAY

BREAKFAST ___________________

LUNCH ___________________

SNACKS ___________________

DINNER ___________________

TUESDAY

BREAKFAST ___________________

LUNCH ___________________

SNACKS ___________________

DINNER ___________________

WEDNESDAY

BREAKFAST ___________________

LUNCH ___________________

SNACKS ___________________

DINNER ___________________

THURSDAY

BREAKFAST ___________________

LUNCH ___________________

SNACKS ___________________

DINNER ___________________

FRIDAY

BREAKFAST ___________________

LUNCH ___________________

SNACKS ___________________

DINNER ___________________

SATURDAY

BREAKFAST ___________________

LUNCH ___________________

SNACKS ___________________

DINNER ___________________

SUNDAY

BREAKFAST ___________________

LUNCH ___________________

SNACKS ___________________

DINNER ___________________

NOTES

____

____

____

____

WEEKLY MEAL PLANNER

DATE:

MONDAY

BREAKFAST ___________________

LUNCH ___________________

SNACKS ___________________

DINNER ___________________

TUESDAY

BREAKFAST ___________________

LUNCH ___________________

SNACKS ___________________

DINNER ___________________

WEDNESDAY

BREAKFAST ___________________

LUNCH ___________________

SNACKS ___________________

DINNER ___________________

THURSDAY

BREAKFAST ___________________

LUNCH ___________________

SNACKS ___________________

DINNER ___________________

FRIDAY

BREAKFAST ___________________

LUNCH ___________________

SNACKS ___________________

DINNER ___________________

SATURDAY

BREAKFAST ___________________

LUNCH ___________________

SNACKS ___________________

DINNER ___________________

SUNDAY

BREAKFAST ___________________

LUNCH ___________________

SNACKS ___________________

DINNER ___________________

NOTES

____

____

____

____

WEEKLY MEAL PLANNER

DATE:

MONDAY

BREAKFAST _______________

LUNCH _______________

SNACKS _______________

DINNER _______________

TUESDAY

BREAKFAST _______________

LUNCH _______________

SNACKS _______________

DINNER _______________

WEDNESDAY

BREAKFAST _______________

LUNCH _______________

SNACKS _______________

DINNER _______________

THURSDAY

BREAKFAST _______________

LUNCH _______________

SNACKS _______________

DINNER _______________

FRIDAY

BREAKFAST _______________

LUNCH _______________

SNACKS _______________

DINNER _______________

SATURDAY

BREAKFAST _______________

LUNCH _______________

SNACKS _______________

DINNER _______________

SUNDAY

BREAKFAST _______________

LUNCH _______________

SNACKS _______________

DINNER _______________

NOTES

____

____

____

____

WEEKLY MEAL PLANNER   DATE:

MONDAY

BREAKFAST ___________________

LUNCH ___________________

SNACKS ___________________

DINNER ___________________

TUESDAY

BREAKFAST ___________________

LUNCH ___________________

SNACKS ___________________

DINNER ___________________

WEDNESDAY

BREAKFAST ___________________

LUNCH ___________________

SNACKS ___________________

DINNER ___________________

THURSDAY

BREAKFAST ___________________

LUNCH ___________________

SNACKS ___________________

DINNER ___________________

FRIDAY

BREAKFAST ___________________

LUNCH ___________________

SNACKS ___________________

DINNER ___________________

SATURDAY

BREAKFAST ___________________

LUNCH ___________________

SNACKS ___________________

DINNER ___________________

SUNDAY

BREAKFAST ___________________

LUNCH ___________________

SNACKS ___________________

DINNER ___________________

NOTES

____

____

____

____

WEEKLY MEAL PLANNER

DATE:

MONDAY

BREAKFAST _______________

LUNCH _______________

SNACKS _______________

DINNER _______________

TUESDAY

BREAKFAST _______________

LUNCH _______________

SNACKS _______________

DINNER _______________

WEDNESDAY

BREAKFAST _______________

LUNCH _______________

SNACKS _______________

DINNER _______________

THURSDAY

BREAKFAST _______________

LUNCH _______________

SNACKS _______________

DINNER _______________

FRIDAY

BREAKFAST _______________

LUNCH _______________

SNACKS _______________

DINNER _______________

SATURDAY

BREAKFAST _______________

LUNCH _______________

SNACKS _______________

DINNER _______________

SUNDAY

BREAKFAST _______________

LUNCH _______________

SNACKS _______________

DINNER _______________

NOTES

____

____

____

____

WEEKLY MEAL PLANNER

DATE:

MONDAY

BREAKFAST _______________

LUNCH _______________

SNACKS _______________

DINNER _______________

TUESDAY

BREAKFAST _______________

LUNCH _______________

SNACKS _______________

DINNER _______________

WEDNESDAY

BREAKFAST _______________

LUNCH _______________

SNACKS _______________

DINNER _______________

THURSDAY

BREAKFAST _______________

LUNCH _______________

SNACKS _______________

DINNER _______________

FRIDAY

BREAKFAST _______________

LUNCH _______________

SNACKS _______________

DINNER _______________

SATURDAY

BREAKFAST _______________

LUNCH _______________

SNACKS _______________

DINNER _______________

SUNDAY

BREAKFAST _______________

LUNCH _______________

SNACKS _______________

DINNER _______________

NOTES

____

____

____

____

WEEKLY MEAL PLANNER

DATE:

MONDAY

BREAKFAST _______________

LUNCH _______________

SNACKS _______________

DINNER _______________

TUESDAY

BREAKFAST _______________

LUNCH _______________

SNACKS _______________

DINNER _______________

WEDNESDAY

BREAKFAST _______________

LUNCH _______________

SNACKS _______________

DINNER _______________

THURSDAY

BREAKFAST _______________

LUNCH _______________

SNACKS _______________

DINNER _______________

FRIDAY

BREAKFAST _______________

LUNCH _______________

SNACKS _______________

DINNER _______________

SATURDAY

BREAKFAST _______________

LUNCH _______________

SNACKS _______________

DINNER _______________

SUNDAY

BREAKFAST _______________

LUNCH _______________

SNACKS _______________

DINNER _______________

NOTES

____

____

____

____

WEEKLY MEAL PLANNER

DATE:

MONDAY

BREAKFAST _______________

LUNCH _______________

SNACKS _______________

DINNER _______________

TUESDAY

BREAKFAST _______________

LUNCH _______________

SNACKS _______________

DINNER _______________

WEDNESDAY

BREAKFAST _______________

LUNCH _______________

SNACKS _______________

DINNER _______________

THURSDAY

BREAKFAST _______________

LUNCH _______________

SNACKS _______________

DINNER _______________

FRIDAY

BREAKFAST _______________

LUNCH _______________

SNACKS _______________

DINNER _______________

SATURDAY

BREAKFAST _______________

LUNCH _______________

SNACKS _______________

DINNER _______________

SUNDAY

BREAKFAST _______________

LUNCH _______________

SNACKS _______________

DINNER _______________

NOTES

____

____

____

____

WEEKLY MEAL PLANNER

DATE:

MONDAY

BREAKFAST ___________________

LUNCH ___________________

SNACKS ___________________

DINNER ___________________

TUESDAY

BREAKFAST ___________________

LUNCH ___________________

SNACKS ___________________

DINNER ___________________

WEDNESDAY

BREAKFAST ___________________

LUNCH ___________________

SNACKS ___________________

DINNER ___________________

THURSDAY

BREAKFAST ___________________

LUNCH ___________________

SNACKS ___________________

DINNER ___________________

FRIDAY

BREAKFAST ___________________

LUNCH ___________________

SNACKS ___________________

DINNER ___________________

SATURDAY

BREAKFAST ___________________

LUNCH ___________________

SNACKS ___________________

DINNER ___________________

SUNDAY

BREAKFAST ___________________

LUNCH ___________________

SNACKS ___________________

DINNER ___________________

NOTES

____

____

____

____

THANK YOU!!!